The Simple Guide to Financial Management Hiring

The Simple Guide to Financial Management Hiring

PENNY M. CROW

M. CHRISTINE KALISH

SHARON Z. GINCHANSKY

MGMA

Medical Group Management Association®

Item: 1025

ISBN: 978-1-56829-691-3

Printed in the United States of America

10 9 8 7 6 5 4 3 2 1

Contents

Purpose of the Hiring Guide

"People are not your most important asset. The right people are." – Jim Collins

The Basics

This book will help you think about hiring in ways you haven't thought about it before. Throughout this book, you will see small icons that will indicate three categories of information.:

	General information that is repeated in each of the hiring guides published by MGMA
	Specific information that is required information for the category of jobs being discussed and is only in this manual.
	These are isolated boxes meant to highlight information like pro tips and best practices.
	Key takeaway summaries are included throughout.

The core information in this guide is focused on the full recruitment cycle, outlined below:

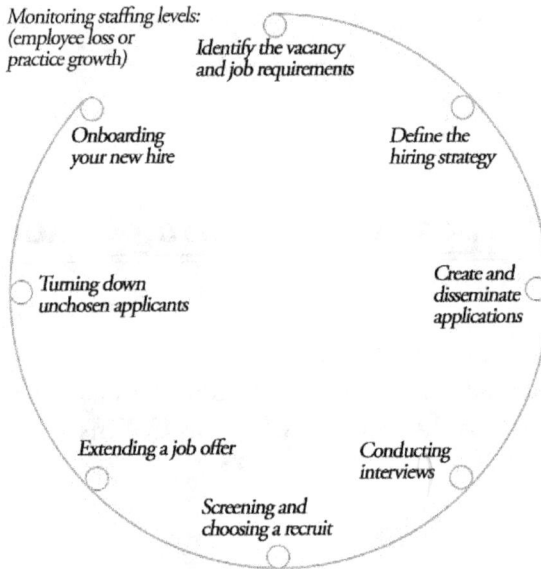

Monitoring staffing levels: (employee loss or practice growth)

Identify the vacancy and job requirements

Onboarding your new hire

Define the hiring strategy

Turning down unchosen applicants

Create and disseminate applications

Extending a job offer

Conducting interviews

Screening and choosing a recruit

Why does a medical practice need a hiring guide?

For many practices, hiring and recruitment is not a full-time, or even regular, activity. This hiring guide is written for everyone who manages staff or might be responsible for tasks involving human resources. This can be a narrow or broad group of resources and can include practice managers, physician-owners, and other staff, such as supervisors, recruiters, interviewers, trainers, compensation managers, HR specialists, legal/compliance coordinators, and researchers.

This guide takes the reader through the entire process from job analysis to description creation and through to hiring and onboarding. While it includes documents, tools, and related job descriptions, the guide is written in such a way that a practice can reference a certain section to focus in on just that information. This manual is tactical and process-oriented, providing step by step instructions for hiring tasks that might not be included in the daily workstream. It outlines the proactive strategies required to define, attract, and retain qualified applicants.

One of the challenges in a medical practice, especially smaller ones with limited resources, is the limited preparation before a vacancy occurs. When the manager receives a two-week notice from someone considered to be a valued or key employee, a couple of things tend to occur. First, the manager thinks they have more time than really exists to replace that employee; second, the manager imagines they might be able to convince the employee to stay. The reality is that the manager must act, and act quickly. Without a clear-cut process that can be immediately executied to begin the recruitment process, the gap for the practice may have nearly-immediate impacts on day-to-day operations. This manual, when used to its maximum benefit, will assist the medical practice in building a base for recruiting, hiring, and retaining staff that will allow the responsiveness and quick pivots required for today's medical practice environment.

This guide addresses the consistent processes and points out those that are specific to the job category in the title. While the rules and regulations for hiring and recruiting may be similar, different job levels and categories present unique challenges along the way. This tool provides tricks, tips, and best-practice ideas to support every size medical organization.

All staff should have access to this tool. Too often, organizations limit human resources and hiring functions to those who supervise, manage, or own the practice. Almost all staff, at one time or another, will be asked to participate in some part of the recruitment and hiring process. This guide also ensures *everyone* follows the appropriate process when bringing new staff into the practice. Additionally, this guide may help employees understand how their job relates to others in the practice. Sharing this information, so employees understand cause and effect, job performance, and the importance of improvement, benefits the entire organization.

Analyzing Medical Practice Staffing

"Time spent on hiring is time well spent." – Robert Half

As much as an organization wants to think that they are proactive about planning for staff changes, too often those plans are set aside when faced with the clear priority to provide excellent care to patients and deliver the associated day-to-day tasks. When a vacancy opens within an organization, the natural inclination is to move forward with filling the position as quickly as possible. The better strategy is to use the vacancy as an opportunity to assess staffing needs and determine if the organization can benefit from doing more than just hiring for the same job. This activity will take more time, but what the practice will gain in the long run by having a well-rounded team cannot be underestimated.

Even before the practice writes or updates a job description, the manager needs to make sure the projected position will meet the needs of the organization. Asking some questions and completing a short analysis will set the baseline for the hiring process and define an order of operations.

The first step is to better understand why there is an opening. What caused the individual to leave the position?

Reasons can include:

- Workload
  - o Real or perceived workload disparities will create disagreements in the practice.
- Personality and fit
  - o Company culture can make or break a team, and team attitude can make or break the culture.
- Managerial issues
  - o People don't leave jobs; they leave managers.
- Compensation
  - o Real or perceived compensation discrepancies create disgruntled employees.
- Training
  - o A practice cannot expect the best from employees if they aren't trained appropriately.
- Personal
  - o Life events and family commitments that are out of the practice's control.
- Career Advancement
  - o It is difficult to provide numerous advancement opportunities in a smaller practice, however, there are different methods of addressing that in order to retain employees.

The practice can determine the answer to these questions through employee interviews and exit interviews—and through observing workflow and the personal interactions. There are tools available to model the process. The key is to keep this simple.

Depending on the answer to the above question, focus on different analyses to determine reasonable changes. Realistically, some things cannot be changed, but the practice may be able to balance that out with the issues that can be changed. For example, if this is about workload, analyze the staffing changes that can be made so the workloads can be distributed more equally and effectively. Small practices are challenged because staff may fill several roles. Roles can grow organically because a staff member may be a stellar performer and won't say no to the extra workload. This easily occurs when services are added that only require a few hours a week, such as scheduling for a part-time provider. The challenge is that workload can grow exponentially and eventually become unmanageable, creating employee dissatisfaction.

Job analysis is usually designed to be work-oriented or worker-oriented. A *work-oriented analysis* results in specific tasks being identified in a typical workday. For example, the receptionist in a small practice may answer phones, schedule appointments, collect monies, and balance the cash drawer. An example of a work-oriented result would be: 'It's time to convert to an electronic process rather than doing a task manually.' A *worker-oriented analysis* focuses on the qualities of the employee, such as knowledge, skills, abilities, and other characteristics (KSAOs) that will contribute to an employee's success in the job.

A ***work-oriented analysis*** results in specific tasks being identified in a typical workday. A ***worker-oriented analysis*** consists of identifying the knowledge, skills, abilities, and other personal attributes that will be important to your practice. It is easier to teach how to complete tasks than it is to make someone fit your culture. Knowing exactly what is needed in a person will make it clearer to identify and hire toward.

Although it is important to hire competent staff, it is equally important that the competent staff also have emotional intelligence, empathy, communication, and other soft skills. This guide discusses how to identify these skills through interviewing techniques. Making poor hiring decisions costs money, creates liability, and results in lost time. Using best practices mitigates these risks. For example, the receptionist needs to be friendly, detail-oriented, reliable, and trustworthy. Whatever job analysis format you use,make sure you are consistent when writing all job descriptions. This information can also be used to determine the salary for a position, training needs, and the performance management process for feedback and evaluation.

Reviewing Relevant Regulations

Before getting into the specifics of the job, it is important to be aware of employment laws that may affect your individual positions. The section below is taken from MGMA's *Job Description Manual for Medical Practices*, 4th Edition (2019).

FLSA (1938)

The **Fair Labor Standards Act of 1938 (FLSA)**, as amended, established minimum wages, equal pay, and overtime; outlawed child labor; and specified record-keeping affecting most full- and part-time employees. One critical part of the law spotlighted in job descriptions is the designation of "exempt" or "nonexempt" job classifications. *Exempt* means that employees holding these jobs are not eligible for overtime pay. These are primarily professional positions. For example, if registered by the state, nurses meet the learned professional exemption and may be classified as exempt if paid on a salary basis of at least $455 per week. Nonexempt employees, such as clerks, are eligible for overtime when they work more than 12 hours in a workday or if they work more than 40 hours in a workweek. The Department of Labor designates which jobs are in which category. The designations do change occasionally. Supervisors should work with an HR specialist to make sure they know which positions are exempt or nonexempt and what that means in terms of overtime pay and other factors.

EPA (1963)

The **Equal Pay Act of 1963 (EPA)** applies to all employers covered by the federal wage and hour law under the Fair Labor Standards Act (see below). It requires that men and women be given equal pay for equal work in the same establishment. The job content, as described in the job description, determines whether jobs are substantially equal.

OSH Act (1970)

The **Occupational Safety and Health Act of 1970 (OSH Act)** established regulations to provide for the health and safety of employees on the job and the Occupational Safety and Health Administration (OSHA). The Act aims to ensure better working conditions by establishing guidelines for employers and employees on work environment conditions. The section in a job description titled "work environment" is a response to this Act and must consider such environmental factors as lighting, workspace, and identifying hazards. Employers must document, track, and report occupational injury and illness trends. Every medical practice should have a safety training plan and conduct such training during orientation and at regular times during employment. Examples of training include courses on body mechanics, infection control, and biohazard protection.

EEO (1972)

The **Equal Employment Opportunity Act of 1972**, referred to as **EEO**, extends the anti-discrimination provisions of Title VII of the 1964 Civil Rights Act. Your lawyer and an HR specialist can help ensure your job descriptions, hiring, and other employment practices comply with the mandate that individuals must be protected against employment discrimination on the basis of race, color, sex, national origin, and religion. It applies to employers with fifteen or more employees. There are two other legal issues to consider. When writing job descriptions, list only the minimum necessary requirements such as education and experience. It is acceptable to note preferred or desirable additional factors, but the emphasis must be on those that are necessary to ensure members of minority groups are not artificially screened out. Also, job descriptions should not state that a job can only be performed by a licensed professional when that is not actually a requirement of the state. For example, states require RNs to be licensed; however, medical assistants are not required to be licensed.

ADA (1990)

The **Americans with Disabilities Act of 1990 (ADA)** prohibits private employers, state and local governments, employment agencies, and labor unions from discriminating against qualified individuals with disabilities in job application procedures, hiring, firing, advancement, compensation, job training, and other aspects of employment. The ADA covers employers with fifteen or more employees. The Act does not protect every disabled person. The person also must be qualified, i.e., an individual who, with or without reasonable accommodation, can perform the essential functions of the job in question. The job description must clearly define those essential job responsibilities, the work environment, the equipment operated, the physical demands, as well as the required knowledge, skills, and abilities. Any person can then be compared with this job profile to ensure the qualification standard is met. HR specialists have the expertise to ensure that you comply with this critical legal regulation.

HIPAA (1996)

The **Health Insurance Portability and Accountability Act of 1996 (HIPAA)** not only focuses on accountability for ensuring patient privacy and confidentiality, it also protects the ability to continue to qualify for health insurance benefits if the employee changes or loses his or her job. It is the patient privacy and confidentiality piece that impacts a job description. Although job descriptions do not need to specify the "need-to-know" level of a job, they frequently emphasize the confidentiality requirement. In all cases, it is important for the supervisor to clearly define a job's confidentiality factors. For example, a clinician caring for a patient needs to know the person's diagnosis; a janitor in the facility does not.

HITECH (2009)

The **Health Information Technology for Economic and Clinical Health Act of 2009 (HITECH)** provides HHS with the authority to establish programs to improve healthcare quality, safety, and efficiency through the promotion of health IT, including electronic health records and private and secure electronic health information exchange. HITECH greatly impacts the need for technological proficiency.

Much of the listed legislation and regulation will affect the medical practice in some way.

Pro Tip: Keeping your eyes on the prize.

- Determine what skillsets can be taught and what must be brought to the table.
- Document the required skillsets.
- Determine traits.
- Determine what is the practice's responsibility to teach, remembering that training is not a one and done.
- Expand the touchpoints for finding competent candidates; this will help you resist the impulse to make the easy hire.
- Be aware that quickly-achieved, short-term relief will almost always equal long-term aggravation.
- Don't forget that it will tend to cost the practice from 3 to 5 times the annual salary if the hire is a mistake.

Conducting a Job Analysis

In larger practices, a consultant may be contracted to complete a job analysis. However, it isn't necessary to bring someone from the outside. The internal hiring manager can use the same tips and tricks for success. First, interview leadership to determine what expectations were set for the job. Next, interview the supervisor of that position, and then, finally, interview the person that actually does the job. It is always educational to see the disconnect between the three descriptions for the same position. This sort of job analysis can help address these discrepancies and provide a decision tool for what the roles and responsibilities of each job should be and, thereby, create a performance standard.

Another way to conduct a job analysis is to observe the current holder of the position and document the tasks being performed. Observing rather than interviewing allows a practice leader to determine if each of these tasks and processes are necessary for today's medical practice. Alternatively, some practices find it useful to have employees complete preprinted questionnaires. And last, but not least, other resources from MGMA may be appropriate for determining the specific tasks and KSAOs necessary for a job. It is important to document all essential functions of the job within the job description. Essential functions are what are considered when an employee requires accommodations made under the ADA. Questions to determine essential job functions include:

- Is this task truly necessary for the job?
- How often does this task have to be done?
- What percentage of time is spent doing this task?
- What happens if the employee doesn't do this task? (Are there consequences?)
- Can the tasks be done differently?
- Can the task be reassigned to someone else?

Now is the time to consider exactly what tasks the position is performing for the team and ask if those tasks:

- are necessary;
- add value; and
- support the core business, which is taking care of the patient.

In addition, consider if technology can be implemented or updated to relieve manual processes. You may find that the position is not really what you thought it was, and so making modifications may ensure retention in that position for the next candidate while boosting the productivity of the entire area or practice. Broken processes and incorrect staffing create significant inefficiencies and cost the practice in quality service, decreasing both patient and employee satisfaction.

If compensation is an issue, first look at the salary or hourly wage relative to the market. Market survey data is available through many sources to determine if the position is being compensated fairly for the work expected. Often this data is difficult to find, particularly when positions are identified differently by each practice. The front desk staff could be patient services representatives or medical receptionist, both doing the same job. When this happens, more analysis is required. Always look in your own backyard to determine if certain positions tend to move frequently, then consider other benefits to encourage retention. In all cases, re-evaluate the budget to see if there is room to increase the salary to be competitive and attract top candidates. Remember that a change for one equals a change for all. Adjusting compensation to keep one employee is never a good idea for the organization.

Take the time to step back and assess workflows to make sure the organizational structure is producing the optimal results. Ask yourself these questions:

- o Are there inefficiencies that can be addressed?
- o Are there processes that are broken?
- o Are there reasons for all tasks being performed?

An individual new to the practice is not accustomed to doing things the usual way, so there is a great opportunity to map out process improvements that can be put into place with a fresh perspective.

Then, always consider personality and fit. Organizational culture, whether the practice is large or small, dictates employee and consequently, patient satisfaction. Be able to understand and communicate the company culture. Know if it's important to have a voice. That will help plan and focus your search. Know who and what you are hiring for.

Wrapping up: Analyzing Medical Practice Staffing

Taking the time to do a thorough analysis of your medical practice staffing is well worth the investment. Before leaping in to quickly replace a departing employee, make sure to gather all the information required to determine the correct staffing solution going forward for the practice. It is also imperative to make sure you understand the market for the role you do wish to hire and that your compensation package is competitive to acquire the quality staff the practice requires.

Key Takeaways

- Reconsider simply recycling the same job description to fill a new vacancy.

- Assess the reasons for the vacancy and make modifications as necessary to make the role as successful as possible.

- Go a step further and see if there are changes that can be made to current processes and workflows to make the organization perform at a higher level.

- Clearly understand your practice culture

Financial Management Roles
within the Medical Practice

"You hire the best people you can possibly find. Then it's up to you to create an environment where great people decide to stay and invest their time."—Rich Lesser

Without argument, healthcare is one of the most complex industries from both an operational and a financial perspective. There are few industries that interface with clients, patients, and stakeholders in the way that healthcare does while providing a myriad of services. There are key market drivers that are creating challenges for medical practices. These include an ever-changing regulatory environment, reimbursement challenges, larger consumer payments, and shrinking margins for the medical practice. In addition, patients recognize the choices they have, including requests for transparency in all aspects of their care. Suddenly providers are faced with new challenges in consumerism, focused on dollars and increased quality of care. These drivers affect the entire practice, including the revenue cycle in financial management and accounting. It is more difficult to maintain operating margins and deliver quality care. This hiring guide focuses on the financial management group of job descriptions.

Depending on the size of the practice and the point of view of leadership, financial management can be assigned responsibility for many functions. For the sake of this discussion, financial management will primarily consist of all accounting, payroll and information technology functions. These staff members provide the oversight for and are the keepers of the data. Overall, they have responsibility to balance the money and the operations with patient care, allowing the providers to do what they do best.

In all practices, financial management professionals have a responsibility and a greater focus on internal controls, risk management, business analytics, with an added higher awareness of systems vulnerability. In smaller practices, financial management can be comprised of one or two people. Often, financial management functions are outsourced to provide checks and balances. Staff can function in different roles, and they may even crossover those roles, depending on the needs of the practice. This guide focuses on the recruitment, hiring, and retention processes for these foundational positions. With the shortage of healthcare professionals predicted in the next couple of years due to an aging population with increased care needs, the growth in the industry indicates a significant potential for financial management professionals. Current revenues means doing more with fewer staff, and the financial management groups have the same issues.

Patients are not typical customers. They are frequently in the middle of a medical crisis and expect and should receive the highest quality of care, often with special handling. Financial management staff may be interacting with patients, in order to find resources for those patients. It is important to understand the skills and attributes needed for these positions. Hiring practices should identify those candidates best qualified to serve in these positions.

As a group, financial management staff require the following skills:

- Stellar communication and customer service skills,
- Industry knowledge and experience,
- High integrity and honesty,
- Ability to multitask and organize, and
- Extreme analytic skills with great attention to detail.

The job descriptions in this category may include:

- Accounting Clerk
- Accounting Manager
- Controller
- Chief Financial Officer
- Payroll Clerk
- Staff Accountant
- Compensation Specialist
- Database Administrator

Let's break this category into functional roles and consider the skills, competencies, and characteristics candidates who will be successful in that job function.

Accounting Manager

Responsibilities and skills could include:

- Providing excellent customer service.
- Performing thorough data collection and entry.
- Acquiring substantial knowledge of accounting systems to allow appropriate monthly close and balance of financial systems.
- Having robust knowledge of HIPAA and privacy practices.
- Be responsible for money management, including budgetary oversight

Their competencies include:

- Possess thorough knowledge of accounting and advancing financial systems.
- Have the ability to balance multiple accounts and entities.
- Can produce clear financial reporting.

- Understands audit processes.
- Understands how the money flows through the practice.

Some of the success characteristics include:

- Attention to detail
- Substantial experience in healthcare
- Service-oriented demeanor
- Excellent communication skills
- High level of discretion
- Ability to interpret financial reports so that non-financial staff will understand

The ability to clearly communicate financial status is a pivotal skill for success in this role. Financial management is really a team sport; it takes the collaboration of the group to close and balance. The team should remain engaged and communicate well.

Compensation Analyst

These are the roles that are directly related to HR functions. Responsibilities and skills could include:

- Managing the payroll system.
- Analyzing current healthcare compensation model and trends and recommend needed changes.
- Guiding the practice in staying compliant with all governmental regulations.

Their competencies include:

- Ability to use compensation and payroll systems.
- Understanding of employment and compensation law.
- Skill in the use of related systems.

Some of the success characteristics include:

- Significant attention to detail
- Ability to interact with all types of stakeholders and personalities

- Pleasant and calm demeanor
- Helpful attitude

The compensation analyst is an important player in the organization. Equitable compensation structures ensure positive outcomes for the practice when recruiting for challenging positions. Analyzing compensation trends is important for the viability of the medical practice in the long-term, for without this information, recruitment will be hampered.

Computer Support Specialist

Many practices might not have the luxury of full-time computer support staff. Whether this is a full-time job or a part of other daily duties around information technology, these responsibilities and skills could include:

- Troubleshooting for all IT-related services, both programs and hardware.
- Maintaining the functionality of all computers and printers.
- Providing education and training to staff.

Their competencies include:

- Communicate well with all staff.
- Listen to provide effective solutions.
- Assess and prioritize urgent problems.
- Understand the importance of working technology to support patient care.
- Extensive knowledge of computer programs and applications.
- Strong knowledge of privacy and security laws and policies.

Some of their success characteristics include:

- Patience
- Attention to detail

- Curiosity
- Desire for continual improvement
- Works independently

These are the staff that provide systems support and technology to allow clinical staff to do what they do best, take care of patients. They provide the data and the analysis to carry out the practice strategy.

Wrapping up: Financial Management Roles

It takes all these related positions to develop, drive, reconcile, and protect financial functions within a medical practice. The complexity of the systems and processes require significant oversight with strategically placed checks and balances. No matter the size of the practice, well trained and experienced financial management and technology staff will protect the interests and sustainability of the organization.

This chapter was a simplistic orientation to the financial management job category within medical practices. A listing of financial management job descriptions is provided in Appendix A. Now that you have a grasp on analyzing staffing and where patient-access roles fit into the medical practice structure, the next chapter will walk through the steps to create a job description.

Key Takeaways

- Soft skills and emotional intelligence are key to successful employees in the financial management job category.
- These positions focus on delivering care while integrating the implications from federal, state, and local regulations.
- Continuing education to keep up with current knowledge and trends in their specialty is generally a requirement for these positions.

Preparing the Job Description

"Under conditions of complexity, not only are checklists a help, they are required for success." - Atul Gawande

Once the cause of the vacancy has been analyzed, it is necessary to determine if the job description is still valid. A job description is a necessary tool that explains how the tasks and duties of a specific job fit into the practice's overall mission and strategic goals. It is important to keep job descriptions up to date, but there is no better time to reassess a position than when it is, or is about to be, vacant.

Writing the Job Description

All job descriptions within the practice should look the same. Standardization and consistency are two of the best defenses in human resource management. Job description methodology continues to be the safest way for employers to have documentation that supports employment decisions and avoids legal issues and complications in hiring, training, and terminating staff. Most importantly, a job description's primary purpose remains stable: to clearly communicate how the employee helps fulfill the goals of the organization. One way to write a job description is to answer the following questions. These answers will design a best-practice-formatted job description. Below are the seventeen core questions to be answered about the position.

Below each question in a gray box is an illustrative (not comprehensive) example response.

1. **What is the job title?**

   - Make the title reflect what the job does. Not only is it important for the employee to understand the title, but a patient reading a name tag needs to be able to determine what this person does. Keeping it simple is always the best naming convention, so be cautious about being creative with titles. Simplicity is one of the best communication tools for the employee and patients to understand the role.

   > **Job title:** Office Manager

2. **What is the job classification?**

   - The Fair Labor Standards (FLSA) is very specific regarding exempt vs. non-exempt positions. *Non-exempt* means that you must pay overtime. Conversely, an *exempt* role is one that is management- or leadership-focused and oversees other staff. Know your state laws and the legal requirements to determine if overtime will be paid on daily or weekly work hours over the standard eight-hour workday. Many practices want to save money by making all their clinical positions exempt to prevent overtime, but the level of responsibility is a primary consideration of job classification. When in doubt, consult an HR professional or attorney for clarification. This conservative approach will protect the practice and the employee from violating IRS rules.

   > **Job classification:** Exempt

3. **To whom does this position report?**

   - This should list the title of the person they will be their supervisor. Keep in mind that the CEO or owner may still report to a board of directors, partners, or investors.
   - Dotted lines between multiple supervisors is not recommended.

   > **Reports to:** Practice Owner

4. **When was the job description last reviewed?**

   - It is helpful to make sure the job is still relevant by dating the job description, which can help trigger a re-assessment if enough time has passed. Nothing can hurt a new employee's satisfaction faster than having the wrong expectations for the job. It is particularly important for executive positions to determine the scope of work executive and the level of expertise needed from the very beginning.

   > **Date:** 08.01.2019

5. **What is the summary of the overall job duties?**

   - This is a summary that allows an employee or candidate to quickly know the expectations.

   > **Summary:** A management position responsible for the daily operations of the medical practice.

6. **What are the essential job responsibilities for this position?**

   - It is important from an employment law defense perspective that essential job responsibilities are listed to determine the applicability of ADA accommodations. The employee will need to be able to successfully complete these specific responsibilities with reasonable accommodations.

- These are the tasks that regardless of physical or mental ability must be done in this individual job.

Essential Job Responsibilities:

- Ensure compliance with current healthcare regulations, medical laws, federal and state laws, and high ethical standards.
- Oversee daily office operations and delegate authority to assigned supervisors.
- Assist supervisors in developing and implementing short- and long-term work plans and objectives for clerical functions.
- Develop guidelines for prioritizing work activities, evaluating effectiveness, and modifying activities as necessary. Ensure that office is staffed appropriately.
- Assist in the recruiting, hiring, orientation, development, and evaluation of clerical staff.
- Establish and maintain an efficient and responsive patient flow system.
- Oversee and approve office supply inventory, ensure that mail is opened and processed, and offices are opened and closed according to procedures.
- Support and uphold established practice policies, procedures, objectives, quality improvement, safety, environmental and infection control, and codes and requirements of accreditation and regulatory agencies.

---

7. What are the competencies (KSAOs) needed?

- It is important for the practice and potential candidate to assess if they are a good fit for each other. This is only possible if the competencies (KSAO) are identified in advance.

- Describe the personal attributes that this employee must have to be successful in this role.

Competencies:

Knowledge

- Knowledge of policies and procedures to manage operations and ensure effective patient care.
- Knowledge of the principles and practices of healthcare administration, fiscal management, and government regulationsand reimbursements.
- Knowledge of Electronic Health Systems.
- Knowledge of Practice Management Systems.
- Knowledge of medical practices, terminology, and reimbursement policies.
- This position requires strong working knowledge of managed care plans, insurance carriers, referrals, and precertification procedures.

Skills

- Skill in exercising a high degree of initiative, judgment, and discretion.
- Skill in analyzing situations accurately and taking effective action.
- Skill in establishing and maintaining effective working relationships.
- Skill in organizing work, delegating and achieving goals and objectives.
- Skill in exercising judgment and discretion in developing, interpreting, and implementing departmental policies and procedures.
- Mastery of spoken and written English.

- Additional languages preferred.
- Possess strong human relations, communication, problem solving, and organizational skills to interact with a variety of customers, payers, vendors, and personnel within and outside the institution.

Abilities:

- Ability to work under pressure, communicate, and present information.
- Ability to read, interpret, and apply clinic policies and procedures.
- Ability to identify problems, recommend solutions, and organize and analyze information.
- Ability to establish priorities and coordinate work activities.
- Ability to work independently and be goal-directed.
- Effectively multitask without compromising quality.
- Ability to comprehend and excel in both verbal and written communication, including proper telephone
- Ability to communicate with individuals and small groups with credibility and confidence.

Other:

- Willingness and desire to maintain regular and acceptable attendance; may be required to work weekend, holiday, or overtime hours.
- Willingness and drive to handle complex, difficult interactions, remain calm under stress, manage emotional situations, display empathy, and maintain positive communication within a rapidly changing/ dynamic environment.

8. Are there any supervisory responsibilities?

- Not all people are leaders and teachers. Supervisory responsibilities include both those attributes. The practice can protect itself by establishing supervision expectations from the beginning. Identify any direct reports.

> **Direct reports:** Business Office Manager, Facilities Manager, Administrative Assistant, Receptionist.

9. **What equipment is does the job require?**

   - Anything that may affect the employee's working conditions such as climate, noise, hours, construction.

   > **Equipment:** Employee expected to be able to use standard office equipment, including computers, fax machines, copiers, printers, telephones, etc.

10. **What is the work environment?**

    - Anything that may affect the employee's working conditions such as climate, noise, hours, construction.

    > **Work environment:** Employee works in a collaborative medical office environment with a private office for confidential conversations. Moderate noise (i.e. business office with computers, phone, and printers, light traffic). Ability to work in a confined area. Ability to sit at a computer terminal for an extended period of time.

11. **What are the physical and mental demands of the essential job functions?**

    - Identify any lifting, bending, sitting, standing, vision, hearing, dexterity and driving requirements.
    - Also include any expected mental demands.

> **Physical and mental demands:**
> - Involves sitting approximately 90% of the day, walking or standing the remainder.
> - Combination of sitting, standing, bending, light lifting and walking.
> - Requires a full range of body motion, including manual and finger dexterity and hand-eye coordination.
> - Lifting up to 20 pounds.
> - Requires corrected vision and hearing to a normal range.
> - Occasional stress from varying demands.

12. **Is this a full time or part time job?**

   - Identify the typical work shift, days and overtime expectations

   > **Position type and expected works hours:** Full time, business hours, Monday through Friday, but occasional evening, holiday, and weekend work. Some flexibility required. Must be available to have a mixed schedule of opening and closing the office and the ability to be flexible with schedule when needed.

13. **Is travel involved?**

   - Candidates need to understand if they are required to travel between clinic locations. Policies will need to be written to outline reimbursement guidelines.
   - List percentage of travel time expected, where the travel occurs, and whether it is overnight travel.

   > **Travel:** Limited travel, primarily local during business hours. Less than 10% of monthly hours.

14. What is the required education and experience?

- Indicate education based on requirements that are job-related and consistent with business necessity. Remember, job descriptions should not state that a job can only be performed by a licensed or certified professional when that is not actually a requirement of the state.

> **Required Education and Experience:**
> - Bachelor's degree.
> - Individuals may also need to complete additional coursework upon hire.
> - Completion of a medical terminology course, or successfully completing one within six months of employment.

15. What is the preferred education and experience?

- Indicate preferred education and experience, but it must relate to this job specifically

> **Preferred Education and Experience:**
> - College-level coursework in healthcare administration preferred.
> - Minimum three years of administrative experience, including at least one year of management experience in healthcare

16. What other eligibility qualifications exist?

- List additional licensure or certification necessary to have this job.

> **Additional eligibility qualifications:**
> - MGMA or PAHCOM certification.

33

17. What other duties as assigned?

- There is no way to identify every task in a practice. This is a general disclaimer statement that catches any other assigned duties.

> Please note this job description is not designed to cover or contain a comprehensive listing of activities, duties or responsibilities that are required of the employee for this job. Duties, responsibilities, and activities may change at any time with or without notice.

18. Include two signature lines.

- The employee and hiring manager should sign the job description and date it.

Putting It All Together

Now that you've answered these questions, you have all the components required to create the final job description. A sample job description for an office manager has been created. Keep in mind this is to be used an an illustrative guide only. This job description and all job descriptions provided in this hiring manual will need to be edited to describe the specific requirements your organization has for that role. Include any information that helps make the duties, responsibilities, and expectations for the role clear.

Job title: Office Manager
Classification: Exempt Reports to Practice Owner Reviewed: 08.01.2019

Summary:
A management position responsible for the daily operations of the medical practice.

Essential Job Responsibilities:

- Enhance patient experiences; optimizing company reputation.
- Ensure compliance with current healthcare regulations, medical laws, federal
  and state laws, and high ethical standards.
- Oversee daily office operations and delegate authority to assigned supervisors.
- Assist supervisors in developing and implementing short- and long-term work plans and objectives for clerical functions.
- Assist supervisors in understanding/implementing clinic policies and procedures.
- Develop guidelines for prioritizing work activities, evaluating effectiveness, and modifying activities as necessary. Ensure that office is staffed appropriately.
- Assist in the recruiting, hiring, orientation, development, and evaluation of clerical staff.
- Establish and maintain an efficient and responsive patient flow system.
- Oversee and approve office supply inventory, ensure that mail is opened and processed, and offices are opened and closed according to procedures.
- Support and uphold established policies, procedures, objectives, quality improvement, safety, environmental and infection control, and codes and requirements of accreditation and regulatory agencies.

Competencies:

Knowledge

- Knowledge of policies and procedures to manage operations and ensure effective patient care.
- Knowledge of the principles and practices of healthcare administration, fiscal management, and government regulations and reimbursements.
- Knowledge of Electronic Health Systems.
- Knowledge of Practice Management Systems.
- Knowledge of medical practices, terminology, and reimbursement policies.
- This position requires strong working knowledge of managed care plans, insurance carriers, referrals, and precertification procedures.

Job title: Office Manager

Skills

- Skill in exercising a high degree of initiative, judgment, and discretion.
- Skill in analyzing situations accurately and taking effective action.
- Skill in establishing and maintaining effective working relationships.
- Skill in organizing work, delegating and achieving goals and objectives.
- Skill in exercising judgment and discretion in developing, interpreting, and implementing departmental policies and procedures.
- Skill in planning and supervising.
- Skill in evaluating the effectiveness of existing methods and procedures.
- Mastery of spoken and written English;

Abilities

- Ability to establish and maintain effective working relationships with other employees and the public.
- Ability to communicate and present information under pressure.
- Ability to read, interpret, and apply clinic policies and procedures.
- Ability to identify problems, recommend solutions, organize and analyze information.
- Ability to establish priorities and coordinate work activities.
- Ability to work independently and be goal-directed.
- Effectively multitask without compromising quality.
- Ability to comprehend and excel in both verbal and written communication, including proper telephone etiquette, face-to-face interactions, and electronic communications.
- Ability to communicate with individuals and small groups with credibility and confidence.

Other

- Willingness and desire to maintain regular and acceptable attendance; may be required to work weekend, holiday, or overtime hours. Must be available to have a mixed schedule of opening and closing the office and the ability to be flexible with schedule when needed.
- Willingness and drive to handle complex, difficult interactions, remain calm under stress, manage emotional situations, display empathy, and maintain positive communication within a rapidly changing/dynamic environment.

Position Type and Expected Works Hours:

Full time, business hours, Monday through Friday, but occasional evening, holiday, and weekend work. Some flexibility required.

Job title: Office Manager

Equipment Operated:

Standard office equipment, including computers, fax
machines, copiers, printers, telephones, etc.

Physical and Mental Demands

- Involves sitting approximately 90% of the day, walking or standing the remainder.
- Combination of sitting, standing, bending, light lifting and walking.
- Requires a full range of body motion including manual and finger dexterity and hand-eye coordination.
- Lifting up to 20 pounds.
- Requires corrected vision and hearing to a normal range.
- Occasional stress from varying demands.

Travel:
- No travel is expected for this position.

Required Education and Experience:

- Bachelor's degree,
- Individuals may also need to complete additional coursework upon hire.
- Completion of a medical terminology course or successful completion within six months of employment.

Preferred Education and Experience:

- College-level coursework in healthcare administration preferred.
- At least one year of healthcare administration experience.

Additional Eligibility Qualifications:
- MGMA, PMI, or PAHCOM certification.

Other Duties:

Please note this job description is not designed to cover or contain
a comprehensive listing of activities, duties or responsibilities that
are required of the employee for this job. Duties, responsibilities
and activities may change at any time with or without notice.

Signatures

This job description has been approved by all levels of management:

Manager_____

Employee signature below constitutes employee's understanding of
the requirements, essential functions and duties of the position.

Employee_____ Date _____

Wrapping up: Preparing the Job Description

This Office Manager job description is simply a road map. A carefully constructed job description identifies what is negotiable and what isn't for this clinical function. When this important stage of hiring is overlooked, it is much easier to compromise what is needed for the position, which can result in a poor hiring decision. Making poor hiring decisions costs the practice money, creates liability, and results in lost time. Using best practices will mitigate these risks.

It is as important for the candidate to assess the practice as vice versa. A well-written job description can be the perfect communication tool. Although the interview is important for a face to face discussion, it is the job description that is setting the tone for the discussion. It is also one of the best defense tools in employment complaints.

The job description helps ensure that the future employee and the practice are a good fit for each other. It sets the expectations from the beginning and can be used for orientation, feedback sessions, and the annual performance review. A good job description protects both the employer and the employee from unexpected surprises.

So, what's next? It is time to recruit to find the right candidate for the right job.

Key Takeaways

- Job descriptions should complement the practice mission.
- Good job descriptions establish the expectations of the candidate, employee, and management.
- It is necessary to know key HR laws when writing job descriptions to protect the practice.

The Recruitment Process Reconsidered

"Hiring the best is your most important task."
Steve Jobs

Recruitment at its core, is a basic, fundamental activity in all businesses. It is a process that if done well will help secure the practice's future. Why is it so important? It's important because it helps solidify the practice's reputation.

Consider this—if you walked into a medical practice for an interview, the front desk was unmanned, they weren't aware you were coming in for an interview, the interview was then conducted haphazardly and unfinished, what would you walk away thinking about that medical practice? Most likely, you would walk away thinking the practice does not know what they are doing, they were disorganized, disorderly, and treated you poorly.

How would you talk about that practice in the future? You, and others, would speak ill of the practice, telling this story possibly years to come. This might just be an interview gone awry and may not be a clear picture of the practice, but the story would linger in a negative way.

How do you rectify this? Using best practices to recruit staff that create the workplace culture you want in your medical practice. If you have recruited properly and filled your open positions with the best fit from a business and culture perspective, your business will thrive.

Satisfied employees create a satisfied patient population, which will create a successful practice, according to studies reported by *Forbes*. A successful practice means there is a likelihood that the practice will continue. Business continuity and continuation is vital, without successful caring individuals who think of your business as their business, your practice won't reach its full potential. This impacts not only the sustainability of your practice but the growth and the revenue overall. Your employees are your first line of customer service, excellent customer service will bring your patients and families back time and again.

The Recruitment Process

The recruitment process, from analysis to onboarding, is a costly endeavor. The process takes time and energy to complete in a manner that acquires the best candidates and the best employee. The costs associated with recruitment are extensive, including the time it takes away from your core business, but it is a requirement.[1] In a series of case studies analyzed by the Center for American Progress, it was found that 'quick hiring' could save an employer up to 50% of the employee's annual salary versus a full recruitment drive with analysis—but that there would be a better than 25% chance that within a year employee turnover would cost the company anywhere from 5% up to 213% of the employee's annual salary[2] This is why hiring has to be executed well the first time around. Besides the financial deterrent associated with recruiting and hiring the wrong employee, there are other impacts that will ripple through your entire business in a number of ways—some that cannot be calculated, including:

- decreased productivity,
- turnover,

---

[1] Bersin, Josh. "Employee Retention Now a Big Issue: Why the Tide has Turned," LinkedIn Influencer, August 16, 2013, https://www.linkedin.com/pulse/20130816200159-131079-employee-retention-now-a-big-issue-why-the-tide-has-turned/

[2] Boushey, Heather and Sarah Jane Glynn. "There Are Significant Business Costs to Replacing Employees," Center for American Progress, November 16, 2012, https://www.americanprogress.org/wp-content/uploads/2012/11/CostofTurnover.pdf

- decreased patients seen,
- delayed service times,
- negative viewpoints from customers and employees,
- not enough resources,
- lower morale,
- gossip, and
- information not shared between staff.

The only way to mitigate these costs is hire right the first time using tried and true methods to bring in the best candidate.

What is your turnover rate?

How many people left your practice last year? (X)

What were the total number of positions last year? (Y)

Divide number who left by the number of positions. (X/Y)

That's your turnover rate—for every role turned over, there is both a replacement cost and a cost to your business for not having that role filled

---

How to start the recruitment process.

After you have completed the analysis and determined your practice's needs, consider both *how* and *where* to recruit.

How will you recruit for this position?

The simplest answer is that recruitment comes from many sources to attract and satisfy diverse candidates. It can also be described as using any way possible that yields the best candidates. Examples of methods include:

- Create a superior hiring package:
    - o   Offer better compensation than the local market.
    - o   Offer better benefits (such as health or 401K).
    - o   Offer better career advancement packages.

- Create a stronger culture fit:
  - Offer a closer knit, more supportive environment.
  - Offer a greater scope of employment-based interests and challenges.
  - Offer ties to the local community.
- Create a better tomorrow:
  - Offer education support.
  - Offer vested interest in the company.
  - Extend expanded benefits (not just health) to include employee families (a matching college fund for kids is a powerful retention tool for top recruits.)
- Create personal satisfaction:
  - Offer challenges tailored to the personality of the recruit.
  - Offer team-based reverse interviews to allow top recruits to "interview" you.
  - Allow for flexibility by allowing the recruit choice in one or more non-key functions (things like local charity drive management or inter-office sports activities).

CAUTION

Using a recruiter or a headhunter is expensive. It can cost in excess of 20% of the annual salary unless you have a retained agreement for the recruiter. Before you hire a recruiter, consider whether or not you can successfully recruit internally.

Where should I recruit from?

There are many places to garner qualified and experienced candidates. The first step is to determine if are you going to recruit for this position yourself without using an agency or a recruiter. If you choose to use a recruiter for this position, confirm the details of the contract. The contract should list and explain the associated costs, such as who has the responsibility to pay for any possible advertising or related out-of-pocket expenses. In addition, the contract should cover

> **Pro Tip:** Ask your current employees for referrals, encourage them to seek out the candidates. Your employees know your workplace, they are well connected, they are your greatest recruiters. For tough to fill roles, incentivize employees with referral bonuses or raffles. Encourage them to post on their social media accounts.

what happens if a candidate applies for the position on their own and is also presented by the recruiter and how to manage previous candidates you've interviewed. It should also address how long the contract period is in place and identify the specific positions for recruitment. Then negotiate who completes the background or licensure verification and references and who your practice works with during the process. These items should be clearly delineated in the contract so you are not haggling or reviewing this after you've found your ideal candidate.

Finding the right candidate on your own is not only possible, but achievable, if you put in the effort. Start by thinking where you want to post the job opening.

The greatest asset you have is your current employee base. Begin by telling your employees the practice has a job opening, then give them a flyer or show them the job posting. Ask your staff for help to fill this job. Be clear with your employees what it is you're looking for in a potential candidate. The more direct you are with your staff, the better the referral will be in the long run. If you need someone who has a specialized degree, tell them. There is nothing worse than having someone referring be told after the fact you were looking for something specific. Don't let your employees put themselves out there with their colleagues or friends only to be embarrassed.

> **Pro Tip:** Look at postings by searching the job title and seeing what others post. This will help you create the best post using keywords and common themes.

Posting an open position is relatively easy now with many little-to-no-cost options. As in all searches, the practice should have a plan to attract the most qualified candidates. Consider postings based on the position, as follows:

- **Create a job posting flyer.** List the who, what, where, when, how, and why of interesting tidbits the candidate will be searching for in their category. Make it appealing, eye catching, and easy to read.
- **Post to job boards like Indeed or ZipRecruiter.** Job boards have low cost models to help small businesses. Indeed also searches for web posts and will link to your job some of the time. Do not count on this, as it does not always happen.
- **Post to LinkedIn.** If your business does not have a LinkedIn account, consider this the ultimate time to start one. Moreover, create one for your practice administrator specifically to post these positions.

Where do you post for the job opening?

- Executive search firms will contact you—make adecision if you wish to do this, if not then proceed with normal recruitment activities .
- Networking—business contacts, community organizations (Rotary Club, Executive Coaches), former business associates.
- Indeed, ZipRecruiter, LinkedIn, Craig's List, local community colleges, local universities/colleges,
- Never underestimate the power of social media and personal relationships for these positions

Pro Tip: When posting for the job, if you want to an easy pre-screen, provide the requirements, such as a certification from HFMA or a CPA.

- **Social media.** Is the practice on social media? If so, use the flyer to post this position with a hyperlink for an email or application process.
- **Local schools.** Local universities and/or colleges are an excellent place to connect with job prospects. Alert the career center and/or professors/teachers in this field that you are hiring.
- **Your website.** This is a great place to sell your own organization. Your patients may have referrals and that will speak volumes about your practice!
- **Networking, local organizations, and affiliations.** Are you a member of local organizations or networking group? Do you attend monthly meetings in your field? These are logical places to post these positions and discuss the opening.

You have candidates, now who do you interview?

Most importantly, you must assess the candidates fairly.

- What should you be looking for?
  - Credentials
    - Be fair and equal—it is important to review all candidates equally to avoid any future concerns.
    - Minimum standards—candidates that do not meet the minimum standards will not be prioritied for interviews.
    - Preferred requirements—if applicants meet the preferred requirements, they will be placed at the top of the list for interviews.
    - Skills required for the position—if an applicant meets all the requested skills, the candidate will go to the top for interviews.
  - Job history
    - Assure the job history reflects the skills need for the posted position. It is important to inquire about gaps in the history.

o Instructions
  ❑ Did the applicant follow instructions properly on how to apply? For example, if you requested a salary history and he/she did not provide one, will you exclude the applicant? Perhaps not, but it is good to know your boundaries and what you're willing to waive. This is very important, because if you waive any for one applicant, you must waive it for all.

o Résumé
  ❑ Was the résumé tailored for your position? If it is a generic résumé, does it meet your needs?

o Initiative
  ❑ Did the applicant take initiative by reaching out to the hiring manager or practice administrator?

o Cover letter
  ❑ Did they send one? Is it specific to the job you are posting?

> **Pro Tip:** Create a form to add on top of each résumé to assess each candidate fairly.
>
> Include the following information:
> - Candidate Name
> - Position Applied For
> - Date
> - Minimum requirements listed
> - Minimum requirements met
> - LVN licensed
> - CPR certified
> - Bilingual
> - Interview date

- o Results-oriented
  - ❏ Are the résumé results oriented to showcase their achievements or is it simply a history? This showcases the applicant's work ethic and interest in success.
- o Growth
  - ❏ Is there a history of being moved up, quick growth, or long history of growth? Is the candidate using your practice for growth or to find a home?
- o Competitor
  - ❏ Do they work for a competitor? If so, perhaps you want to interview to get a clearer understanding of the competitor's landscape.

The Application Process

You have now narrowed down your top candidates to interview. The final step in the recruitment process is having an application process that will help you and the candidate carefully discern if offering the position and having it accepted is the right choice for everyone. To best do that, you need to make sure you have an application process that gathers all the pertinent information required.

Do you need an application and a résumé for each applicant?

Absolutely, yes. The résumé is different from an application. The application is a legal document that includes a variety of items that showcase a chronological history of work history, education and skills. Before you interview the candidate, you must have information on each applicant for legal purposes. A résumé is something you will want to have, but it is imperative to have the candidate complete an application.

This is a two-part step that helps the practice get information standardized. All résumés are different and unique to help a candidate stand out to the employer. The application is an equalizer, so all candidates will be judged equally. It gives information about the applicant's background that is not on the résumé. Moreover, the application requires a signature at the end, acknowledging various legal aspects of the interview process. The process allows for more protection for the practice as well.

How do you create an application?

If the practice has a computer-based applicant tracking program, there is a good chance there is an online application process associated with it. Check your system and provider to determine if this is an option. If it is not, there are many samples on the internet to create your own application. The key components[3] to include are as follows:

- Practice name, address, and phone number or use company letterhead
- Applicant's legal name, address, phone number, and email
- Are you eligible to work in the United States? Yes | No
- Are you at least 18 years or older? (If no, you may be required to provide authorization to work.) Yes | No
- Have you ever been terminated from employment or asked to resign by an employer? Yes | No
  - *If yes,* please provide company names and details
- Work History (chronological order with start and end dates) with supervisor name and contact phone number or email along with reason left the employment
- Criminal history
- Salary history
- Educational background
- Preferred schedule (give specific boxes with available day/time combinations)
- How did you hear about us? Walk In | Advertisement | Referral | Other
- Have you ever worked for this company before?
- Do you know anyone who works for our company?
- Reference Listing (3) name, phone number, email, company

---

[3] Society for Human Resource Management (SHRM) example

- Legal signatures (signing that they understand the practice is an at-will employer)
- It is very important to include something like the following disclosure statement, which the applicant should sign separately:

Please read carefully before signing.

[Practice Name] is an equal opportunity employer. [Practice Name] does not discriminate in employment on account of race, color, religion, national origin, citizenship status, ancestry, age, sex (including sexual harassment), sexual orientation, marital status, physical or mental disability, military status or unfavorable discharge from military service.

I understand that neither the completion of this application nor any other part of my consideration for employment establishes any obligation for [Practice Name] to hire me. If I am hired, I understand that either [Practice Name] or I can terminate my employment at any time and for any reason, with or without cause and without prior notice. I understand that no representative of [Practice Name] has the authority to make any assurance to the contrary.

I attest with my signature below that I have given to [Practice Name] true and complete information on this application. No requested information has been concealed. I authorize [Practice Name] to contact references provided for employment reference checks. If any information I have provided is untrue, or if I have concealed material information, I understand that this will constitute cause for the denial of employment or immediate dismissal.

Date _____ Signature _____

THIS APPLICATION IS VALID ONLY FOR 60 DAYS FROM THE DATE SIGNED/DATED ABOVE.

Wrapping up: Recruitment

Mindful recruitment strategies will be one of the most important commitments you can make to growing the future of your practice culture, teams, and organization. Find ways to introduce consistency into your approach and maximize the potential of your networks and connections. An improved recruitment process can be one of those opportunities where a practice can reap the rewards a seasoned practice manager's persistence and dedication can bring to a problem.

Key Takeaways

- Being consistent in your approach and methodical in your processes will significantly benefit you and your practice or organization in the long run.
- Careful preparation will help you hire the correct candidate.
- A careful application process is the best way to make the seeds of your recruitment efforts bear fruit.

Designing a Hiring Process

"You don't hire for skills, hire for attitude. You can always teach skills." – Simon Sinek

After all the upfront time and energy you took to prepare for the recruitment and application processes, it is time to find the right candidate through a carefully crafted hiring process. This process has a series of fundamental steps, which will be outlined below. By implementing a few best practices, you will be able to refine your process and find the right candidate for your practice.

The Hiring Process

Keep in mind, as you build out your hiring process, that the first and foremost concern is to create a candidate experience that is positive. Aside from any damage the practice's reputation might suffer from word getting around about a poor interview experience, your ideal result is a candidate who very much wants to work for your practice. A carefully crafted process will provide the required structure when the impacts of day-to-day operations might normally cause you to forward in ways that are not ideal.

There will be some steps that will need to be altered depending upon the role being filled. One of those steps is the candidate interview. It can be helpful to have a pre-determined strategy for different types of roles, so that when you have an opening for that type of role, you are clear about your intended interviewing strategy. Similarly, having a pool of questions for those interviews available based on the role will help shorten the time required to prepare for interviews. See Appendix B for some suggested questions based on roles outlined in this hiring manual. Here is a broad outline of the hiring process:

1. Ensure that an applicant tracking system is in place and being followed.

2. Select an interview strategy if one is not already in place.

3. Identify important questions.

4. Prepare the total compensation calculation.

5. Outline ways to understand candidates' alignment with the practice culture.

6. Conduct phone and face-to-face interviews prioritized by candidates who are the best fit for the identified role requirements.

7. Make an offer.

8. Perform pre-employment requirement checks.

9. Communicate with declined applicants.

10. Onboard the new hire.

11. Have a process for reviewing the new hire during the probationary period.

Tracking System for Applicant Information

Most small practices and even larger ones will not have a tracking mechanism or system for tracking the applicants. Some payroll systems have this built in, so make sure to check with your payroll provider. If you don't have an automated system, an Excel spreadsheet is the easiest way track. If you don't have an Excel spreadsheet, you can create something similar in Word or by hand. The spreadsheet/document should include the applicant's name, application date, referred by, interview dates, including any phone interviews. If you have a much larger practice, you may want to invest in an applicant flow tracking system that tracks

Pro Tip: Retain all applicant information collected and any related hiring notes for a minimum of 3 years.

Preserve the application information for candidates within a personnel file in a locked filed cabinet behind a locking office door. Personnel file retention regulations vary from state-to-state, so check local/state laws for requirements.

applicants anonymously to help ensure no discrimination has taken place. You will also want to have an organized system for keeping all documents related to the hiring process in a secure location.

No matter how well you think it went, you still might receive a call from the EEOC (Equal Employment Opportunity Commission), the Department of Fair Employment and Housing (DFEH), or directly from a lawyer. This is where having your tracking and documentation in place as you go into the process will help you afterwards. Keep in mind, however, that it is not unusual for the EEOC or DFEH simply to be confirming information they have received. Or they may have an anonymous tip that the practice discriminates against a particular group. This is the moment when you take a *deep breath*, grab your hiring notes, your references, any information you pulled, whatever you did to interview and ultimately fill the position. Anything related from the general period of time when you hired that position should be your focus as you prepare to respond to the complaint.

If you receive a formal complaint, contact an HR consultant or a lawyer before answering the complaint. Time is of the essence. While this may be scary or nerve-wracking, do not delay, as there are specific timeframes for response associated with any complaint.

Considerations for small practices vs large practices

The information needed during a governmental review or if a lawsuit should arise is no different. The size of the organization will only come into play in order to determine if your practice is required to meet additional employment standards. The first magic number is 50; the second is 100. If you have fewer than 50 employees, there is some leeway with the requirements of employment laws. However, you must still treat every applicant with respect and dignity, no matter the size of your practice.

Select the Interviewing Strategy

First, determine the best approach to the interview for the particular role that is being filled. Interview strategies are not a one-size-fits-all decision. Some things to consider to select an interviewing strategy:

Who participates in the interviews?

The default choices tend to be the hiring manager or an HR specialist. Some practices opt to have a couple of interviews with different focuses: an HR specialist narrows down the field, then the hiring manager, then a peer or team member. Another alternative to consider would be a team-based approach. Particularly when roles are tightly embedded in a team-based, collaborative culture, the greatest way to accomplish a successful hire is a group interview. These can offer great insight about the team, the role, and the candidate.

Provide the interviewing team with the job description and meet with them to develop the agenda for the interview and an agreed-upon list of questions. Particularly for staff who have little experience interviewing candidates, thinking through the role, what sort of questions to ask, and who should ask them can help them think more thoroughly about what sort of skills and traits they should be looking for in the interview. It will also give you an opportunity to inform them about appropriate interviewing standards and techniques, and confirm the proposed questions conform to best practices (see the "Formulate the Questions" section of this chapter).

Adding a new team member to any group, can be a stressful and time-consuming. Ensure that the candidate's personality, communication style, and mannerisms will fit with the existing staff. Be cautious that individual nuances are not disguising discrimination but

> **Pro Tip:** A phone screening can be a more casual interview; however, there should always be a specific list of questions to structure the interview and provide ease of comparison. Those questions can include:
>
> - Where have you worked?
> - Why are you interested in working for our practice?
> - What type of job title, work schedule, and salary are you looking for in this role?
> - What is prompting the search for a new role?
> - When can you start?
> - What would you say was your proudest work accomplishment?
> - Do you have any questions I can answer?
>
> Phone interviews will usually last from 15 to 30 minutes, depending on the role.

do ensure that the candidate is a complement to the existing staff and is the best fit for your patients. There should be enough similarities that colleagues have things in common, but not so much similarity that the practice loses the benefit of diversity. Team interviews are a great way to experience this fit and discern if the desired synergy is observed.

Use phone interviews to screen applicants

Always complete a phone interview before inviting candidates to your office. An in-person interview takes time, perhaps time that is not available since there is an opening. Conducting a phone interview allows the hiring manager or HR specialist to get a feel for the candidate before committing the time and resourcces to a face-to-face interview. It also allows the for the opportunity to rank applicants to guide the decision on who to invite for the in-person appointments. Phone interviews should be quick confirmations of basic details and a short information-gathering session in order to decide about inviting for an interview. If you've conducted the phone screening and you're not sure if the applicant should come in, let the candidate know you'll be in touch at a later date as you determine the interview schedules.

Take full advantage of the in-person interview

Creating a workplace interview that is positive is similar to creating a practice a patient will want to visit. Below is a possible scenario for setting up the interview for success:

- Invite the applicant to sit down and provide someplace they can wait comfortably. If there is going to be a delay that is any longer than 10 minutes, explain why and thank them for waiting.
- Offer a beverage.
- Provide the candidate with an interview schedule.
- You body language should be relaxed yet energetic. If you are busy and harried, the applicant will feel unwanted or an imposition.
- Treat the candidate respectfully with:
    o Direct eye contact
    o A firm handshake
    o A warm , welcoming smile
- When you invite the applicant into the interview room, make it clear where he or she should sit.
- Give the applicant a tour of the facility, which is an exercise that is useful to you and the applicant, as it is an opportunity to gauge how they fit in the practice environment.)

Formulate the Questions

You will want to prepare a number of questions in advance. Keeping a core list of questions you ask each applicant will ensure uniformity and make later comparisons more equitable. Consider asking behavior-

Pro Tip: There are a few simple best practices for face-to-face interview.

- Do *not* write on the applicant's résumé or application; use a pre-filled out paper to attach to the résumé/application.
- Give applicants a tour of the practice. Look for social or normal cues to determine if they have solid customer service skills and will be a good steward for the organization (e.g., o they make eye contact with the employees and with the patients. Do they pick up trash in the hallway? Do they converse while walking them around? Do they stop for conversation with people?)
- In an interview, it is okay for you to be quiet. Allow the applicant to add more to your question and their answer. If their answer is short, encourage them to tell you more.

based questions that can show you the character of candidates: how they will work and integrate into the culture of the practice. The key is to get to an understanding of how a possible candidate will relate to and solve situations with patients and other staff. The best practice for interviewing is to ask open-ended, conversational questions.

A sampling of open-ended questions includes:

- Please tell me about your career and your background.
- What do you know about this practice?
- What makes you the right candidate for this role?
- After walking the practice, what immediately would you want to change?

Some example scenario-based and behavior-based questions

- Tell me about difficulties you experienced in your last position.
- Describe what work environment makes you your most successful.
- What would you change about your last work environment?
- What do you want me to remember about you after this interview?
- Is there anything else I should know about you and your work history or possible work here?

The questions to never, never ask . . . ever

There are many questions that are inappropriate and unlawful to ask while in an interview. Generally, these are questions that pertain to a person's protected class. A protected class is a group of people qualified for special protection by a law, policy, or similar authority. Overall, it is best to avoid questions that are about gender, color, religion, national origin, gender identity, sexual orientation, political affiliation, family status, disability, or the like. These are questions that, if asked, may open up potential for a discriminatory filing or lawsuit.

A sampling of questions that you should *not ask* are listed below. This is *not* a comprehensive list.

DO NOT ASK
Are you married?
Do you plan to have kids?
What does your spouse do?
Where did you grow up?
What year were you born?
Do you have any bankruptcies?
Have you ever filed a worker's compensation claim?
Have you been injured at work before?
Do you normally wear your hair that way?

DO NOT ASK
Do you have a cane you will use when at the office?
How will you manage the wheelchair in the hallway?
If you got the job, how do you get to work?
Who did you vote for?
Are you a Republican or a Democrat?

Things to share about the practice

The interview process is not only a time for the practice to learn about the candidate, it is also a good time to make sure the candidate understands things about practice and organization standards, policies, and procedures. For example, some clinics don't pay mileage if the person travels straight from their home to the alternate clinic but will pay the standard reimbursement rate if change in location occurs during the day. This expectation should be communicated with the candidate during the interviewing stage. Anything that might be an unpleasant surprise on either side including restrictions on paid time off around holidays, dress code standards, or any other concerns the practice has had to manage in the past should be shared. Keeping a list of these items and sharing them with all applicants will protect the practice from the risk of complaints or litigation.

You've Made a Decision

You've done all the hard work and invested considerable effort into finding just the right person for the role and you now have a candidate you would like to bring onto the team. Now what? It is important at this point for the practice to follow the same hiring practices for each new hire, no matter the role. Implementing a few best-practices steps can go a long way in protecting the practice and providing the candidate the fair and equal opportunity they deserve. You may be eager to go ahead and extend an offer and close the deal, but make all final employment decisions contingent upon your all due-diligence verifications, including background checks, OIG clearance, drug screen, education verification, and skills checks.

> **Pro Tip:** What to ask during a reference check:
>
> - Verify candidate's employment dates, title, salary (they may not give to you).
> - Ask if the person re-hirable.
> - Ask for their overall impression of the candidate.
> - Inquire if there is anything specific you should know about this candidate.
>
> **CAUTION:** Making a hiring decision based purely on one person's reference-call responses could trigger a complaint if the candidate is not hired.

Reference Checks

It is a good idea to call the candidate's references before making an offer. The candidate should consent to you contacting at least three references. References should consist of former employers, supervisors, or colleagues. Reference questions should be standardized. You should ask each person the same questions and then document the answers in the same way. It is important to confirm dates of employment, job title, duties performed, and reason for separation. Remember that while a former employer can say anything that is factual and accurate, what qualifies as factual and accurate can be difficult to prove. Concern over lawsuits causes many former employers to only confirm position, attached salary, and the dates of employment. Despite this, always ask if there is anything they would like to specifically share with you about the candidate.

> **CAUTION:** Do not disclose specific information the references shared with you if the reference is negative. This is confidential.

Document each call or email for the personnel file. Best practice is to have at least two references checked, previous employment or professional references. In some scenarios, a personal reference may be used, but this would be for an entry-level position or someone with little to no work experience. Whatever information is shared should be between you and the reference provider. It should not be shared with the candidate. Reference check are an excellent first line of defense that may protect your organization from having to endure the pain and costs of a bad hire.

Unfortunately, there are many candidates who are either blatantly dishonest or embellish the truth. It is important to fact check information presented by the candidate. You can use social media as a reference point; however, the practice should have policies around the use of this information. The policies will protect the organization, particularly if the social media research shows that the potential candidate belongs to a protected class. Under no circumstances can a person's class or right to free speech be violated or perceived to be violated in preventing them to be considered for a position. While it may be appealing to check on candidates to confirm they would represent your practice well on social media, unless your policies are explicit, acting upon this information may expose the practice to risks.

CAUTION:

Conducting any type of background check before a formal offer is made to the candidate is not appropriate. Do not ask candidates for any identity-related information (e.g., Social Security, previous names, aliases, etc.) without first making an offer.

Total Compensation

The explanation of compensation can be a difficult conversation, so be prepared before making an offer to paint this complete picture. Particularly if the applicant is in a role with labor pool shortages, it will be that much more important to explain the total compensation for the position. *Total compensation* includes all monies the employee will make in this role, including annualized salary, benefits, vacation time value, 401(k) investments, and educational benefits. This is the opportunity for the practice to show the prospective employee what they will fully earn during their employment on an annual basis.

This matters significantly to an employee, as it is their total picture of what they will earn, in salary as well as benefits. It may be useful for some practices to prepare a "Total Compensation Statement" they can provide to the employee to illustrate the true value of working for the practice. The more detailed information, the more beneficial it will be to the potential employee.

You may want to include the following items in a total compensation statement:

- Annualized pay
  - If position is hourly, take the hourly rate x 2080 to get this annualized number.
- Medical benefits
  - Include the amount paid by the employee *and* the employer contribution.
- Flexible spending account
  - Include details on how this is implemented.
- Paid leave
  - List all vacation/sick/PTO, holidays, personal days, floating holidays, or whatever else is offered.
- Volunteer opportunities
  - Describe the volunteer program and recent or near-future projects.
- Disability insurance
  - Short or long term
- Life insurance
  - If paid by the practice, show figures.
- Employee Assistance Program
- Educational Assistance or Tuition Reimbursement
  - Annual amount
- Retirement
  - 401(k) (include any matching).
- Career pathway or advancement

Offer Phone Call Example

Hello. This is _____ from _____. It was a pleasure meeting you and learning about you. After careful consideration we have decided we'd like to offer you the position of _____. The position would pay $_____ per hour, and we'd like you to start on _____. This offer is contingent upon you meeting a number of pre-employment requirements, including a drug screen, criminal background check, and education verification. If you are still interested in the position, we will send you an offer letter and will need some additional information.

Employment Offers and Offer Letters

Following satisfactory reference checks and a confirmed calculation of total compensation, you've reached the decision to extend an offer of employment. What is next? And how is it conducted? The simplest communication method and a best practice is to call the candidate directly and make a verbal offer.

Written offers of employment—contingent offers

The best practice for any type of employment offer, once a verbal offer is accepted, is to make a formal offer in writing. This is done in order to clarify what is being offered, what the pre-employment requirements are prior to the start date, and what the compensation, benefits, and perks for the position are. The letter should explain the offer is contingent upon satisfactory results returned for your practice's pre-employment requirements. The letter should also cover the hourly salary, paydays, supervisor information, benefit information, the start date(s) of those benefits, and who to contact for more benefits information. It should relay information about orientation, training details, schedule, and any other details that will help the new hire feel ready to go when they walk in the practice door on their first day.

Pre-employment Requirements

Every practice, no matter its size, should have a comprehensive list of pre-employment verifications that are performed before the hire is finalized. The practice will need to clearly communicate with the new hire that their employment offer is contingent on the results of those verifications.

Criminal background checks

Background checks are valubale source of protection for your organization. Although the process will cost money, it is minimal compared to what the unknown can cost. Candidates must consent to their background checks and provide their Social Security number, any previous names or aliases, and the names of counties that are applicable based on the candidate's previous residences. The general rule is to review the past 7 years of criminal history.

A reputable background check company should be able to advise you as to what your state/county/local ordinances allow for background checks. The company you have engaged should be able to guide you and recommend what is a best practice for your organization. If they are unsure or cannot provide what you believe to be credible information, move on to a new company. If you try using an internet search firm without customer service, you will most likely not get the type of background check that will satisfy the due diligence standards you and your practice would require. This type of search will yield simple and basic information that will not pass muster in a state or federal survey.

Pre-employment background checks must be administered in compliance with all federal, state, and local laws and all candidates must be treated equally. Decisions for employment cannot be based on a person's race, national origin, color, sex, religion, disability, genetic information, gender identity, ethnicity, political affiliation, or age. For more specific information, refer to the EEOC website.[1] Keep in mind that a criminal background does not automatically eliminate someone from a job. Make sure that you are not discriminating when considering this information. Sometimes the circumstances may influence your decision of the applicability of this information. If you are unsure about

---

[1] https://www.eeoc.gov/eeoc/publications/background_checks_employers.cfm

a candidate's background, it is best to seek out professional human resources consulting or legal advice.

Regardless of the background check results, treat the candidate with respect by keeping information private and confidential. This information is not intended to be shared with the general office population and should be kept in locked and secured files. This information should only be discarded by shredding the information and should not be disposed of in the regular waste basket. Just as a patient's information is considered private and confidential, the practice should protect any candidate and employee's private information.

HHS OIG clearance

Many background check companies will provide, as part of the standard healthcare background check, the U.S. Department of Health and Human Services Office of Inspector General (HHS OIG)'s listing to confirm the candidate is not on the List of Excluded Individuals/ Entities (LEIE), also known as *the exclusion list*. This is mandatory for clinical personnel and a choice for other personnel, however, best practice says conduct this check for all potential employees. The OIG has the authority to exclude individual from federally funded healthcare programs for a variety of reasons, including a conviction for fraud.[2] This includes any pending investigations being conducted by the OIG. If the background company you contract with does not do this, you must do this prior to day one, but after the contingent offer has been made. Any company or person who hires an individual on the list may be subject to civil monetary penalties. Complete this search yourself by visiting the OIG website as listed below and typing in the candidate's name. Take caution—many people have the same names; it is important to confirm identity when withdrawing a job offer.

Illicit drug screening

Many states require a pre-employment drug screen of all healthcare staff. Make sure to check local and state laws. Again, this is done post-

---

[2] https://oig.hhs.gov/exclusions/index.asp

offer and completed once an employment offer is made. Consent is required to conduct the pre-employment drug screen. Choose a vendor that specializes in pre-employment exams. It is best practice for the candidate to have one attempt for the urine drug screen. In other words, if candidates miss the scheduled appointment, they would automatically be disqualified as an employee of the organization.

Skills checks

If a specific skill has been identified in the job description, it is necessary to validate the information is true. This is precisely why a reference check is important. It gives an opportunity to confirm with a prior employer. If it is a new graduate, the instructor or a clinical site supervisor can be one of the references. If it is a technical skill or language competency, quizzes, assessments, or demonstration may provide the confirmation needed. This will be further reviewed in the section in the chapter on orientation and onboarding of personnel. A new hire will need to demonstrate competency in front of a supervisor or peer. This confirmation should be done prior to a new employee working independently without supervision.

Education, licensure, and certifications verification

All job offers should be made as contingent upon verification of education, licensure, and certification status. In recent years, news stories have reported that prestigious leaders of organizations have falsely claimed to hold degrees required for the positions they were holding. Unfortunately, it happens. To protect the organization, make sure to validate education, training, licensure, and/or certifications via the university, trade school, professional association, or state board conferring the credential. Ultimately, it is the leader's responsibility to ensure that the patients are being seen by qualified individuals.

It is essential to confirm all credentials after the offer, but prior to first day, in order to confirm the applicant's résumé is accurate. While you wouldn't expect a well-respected member of your community to not have an accurate résumé, you would be surprised by the percentage of people who do not put the correct information on their résumé. Confirming credentials differs for each role or position category. Larger organizations may use a service to confirm and validate, but smaller practices will usually complete it by phone or online. Either method works as long as it is completed and documented.

Specifically, for administrative positions, credentials may include:

- Degrees
  - o Doctorate in business or public health
  - o Master's degree in health services administration, business, public administration, health informaiton management, or public health
  - o Bachelor's degree
- Licensure and credentials
  - o CPA for accountants
  - o SHRM for human resources managers
  - o CMPE, CMM, CMOM certifications for practice managers
  - o RHIA, RHIT certifications for health information professionals
- Published information or articles

What if the candidate does not meet the requirements?

Not all candidates will pass the pre-employment requirements. When this happens, it is challenging being the person who must rescind the job offer. The cleanest way to do this is to contact the candidate via phone and explain to them in a concise manner that the pre-employment requirements were not met. Tell them that you're very sorry, but you must rescind the offer, and you wish them the best of luck. Although the candidate will usually have some idea they have issues that might identified during pre-employment screening, it is not unusual for the candidate to nonetheless want specific information. If you utilize a company to complete the background check, you can refer them directly to that company. If you completed the background check yourself, you can share the information you discovered.

Occasionally, the information discovered during a pre-employment screening is false or unsubstantiated, e.g., the OIG has multiple similar names or perhaps the drug screen results are inconclusive. When there are questionable results from any of the pre-employment screening, it is recommended to contact the candidate and explain the situation. This gives candidates an opportunity to explain or rectify any issues identified. This is perfectly acceptable. The key is to provide a timeframe within which candidates must resolve the issues or discrepancies. Your position cannot remain open indefinitely. It is best to give the candidate a two-week period or 10 business days to resolve the issue or the offer is rescinded.

Declining other applicants

Many businesses fail to contact other interviewed candidates. It is a part of the process that no one, even the most skilled professional, wants to do. You are relaying a rejection to the candidate, which is difficult both to offer and receive. It is an uncomfortable but key part to closing out the hiring process. The best course of action is to contact each candidate via phone. The hiring manager or HR representative completing the search should contact the face-to-face candidates once the other candidate has passed all contingencies on their employment.

Onboarding Completes the Hiring Process

Onboarding is the time to bring the new employee into your organization, and it involves new hire orientation, training, and the probationary period. It is the opportunity not only to teach the job but

> **Pro Tip:** On an annual basis, all practice employees should be screened against the HHS OIG exclusion list, as this information does change. A suggested process is to run these names, print the results, and place them in a binder or a folder labeled "List of Excluded Individuals Screening for [YEAR]."

> **Pro Tip:** Calculating the onboarding costs per hire
>
> 1. Total pre-employment screening costs per candidate .
> 2. Number of hours to orient and train multiplied by the hourly rate of the trainer
> 3. Number of hours to orient and train multiplied by the hourly rate of the new hire.
> 4. Advertising costs (if any)
>
> Total re-employment screening costs = $85
> Trainer time = $25 x 15 hours = $375
> New hire time $15 x 15 hours = $225
> Advertising costs = $75
> _____
> **Total = $760**
>
> *This is an incredibly modest and conservative number.*

to assimilate the new hire into the practice culture. This is the time to assess their skills hands-on and give them the opportunity to receive the benefit of having supervisor or peer training and guidance. Onboarding is the final piece of the puzzle to having a full-fledged successful member of your team. Proper onboarding is costly; it requires even more effort and time than recruitment. It may be tempting to reduce or eliminate it. But keep in mind that according to the Society for Human Resources Management (SHRM), 69% of employees are more likely to stay with a company for three years if they experienced great onboarding.[3] The majority of employees fail in the first 90-days of employment due to poor onboarding. A survey conducted by Allied Workforce Mobility discovered that companies lose 25% of all new employees within the first year.[4]

---

[3] Maurer, Roy. 2015, April 15. *Onboarding Key to Retaining, Engaging Talent.* Retrieved from   https://www.shrm.org/resourcesandtools/hr-topics/talent-acquisition/pages/onboarding-key-retaining-engaging-talent.aspx.

[4] Allied Workforce Mobility Survey. 2012, March. Retrieved from http://hriq.allied.com/pdfs/AlliedWorkforceMobilitySurvey.pdf.

Make sure to have made all the arrangements and generated the necessary materials to properly onboard the new hire, including employee handbooks, training schedules, peer mentors information, before the new hire's first day. No one benefits from a last-minute scramble added to the already challenging practice environment. Take the time to discuss the onboarding process experience with employees once they complete the probationary stage and be prepared to implement improvements based on that feedback.

Probationary Period

A probationary period is the time the practice has determined is the training period required for the new employee to be successful in that role. A probationary period is generally 90-days. However, this does not mean you simply terminate the employee if they aren't doing a good job. That is not the intention of the probationary period. From day one of the probationary period, the practice should invest in training, assessing, and providing active feedback on the work product of the new employee. It is the supervisor's responsibility to accurately train and develop the new employee. The supervisor should supervise this employee by giving them the tools to be successful, answer questions, follow up on the day's work, and check in every day/week/month to assure the new employee understands and is completing their job assignments properly. The new employee should not at any time be wondering how they are doing in their new job; the supervisor must communicate this on at least a weekly basis, if not daily.

Be prepared for the new hire to struggle at points. It can be helpful to assign a peer mentor if possible or find another way to provide support.Not only will the new hire need support, but the staff will also be adjusting to a new teammate during this period.

Wrapping up: Hiring

The hiring process is the last chance for the candidate and the practice to determine mutual fit. Does the candidate fit the role as far as knowledge, skills, abilities, and attitude? Does the candidate fit with the team and practice culture? Is the role going to be the right one for the candidate?

Answering these key questions is pivotal to the success of the hire, the success of the team, and the success of the practice going forward.

Key Takeaways

- Create a positive candidate experience.
- There are many regulations around the hiring process. Be sure everyone involved has been educated on them, and the practices policies designed to mitigate risk. Don't hesitate to consult an HR specialist.
- Don't waste all the hiring effort by failing to properly train and onboard the new hire. A sink or swim philosophy is not goingn to create success for the new hire or the practice.

Summary

"Hiring people is a form of investing. You have to do your research and make sure you're spending your resources on the right pick." – Warren Buffett

The most important outcome of careful hiring processes is to have an employee base that shares the vision the leadership has for the practice. These employees will represent the practice for a long time. Keep the following points in mind:

- Treat everyone equally and fairly.
- Do not rush the hiring process.
- Prepare the new employee for success with a careful onboarding process.

Hopefully, hiring is not an everyday occurrence in your medical practice. But when it becomes necessary, this guide is available to help remind about best practices. In addition, it will help the practice be more prepared to place the right resources at the right time. Falling short in the hiring process will only lead to turnover in the position and may well have an effect throughout the entire organization. Healthcare is about delivering quality care to patients. Let's put the right people in the right place for the right reasons.

"Always treat your employees exactly as you want them to treat your best customers." – Stephen Covey

Appendix A:
Job Descriptions

Job Title: Accounting Clerk

Department: Administration
Immediate Supervisor Title: Practice Administrator
Job Supervisory Responsibilities: None

General Summary:

A non-clinical position responsible for accounting functions and transactions.

Essential Job Responsibilities:

- Assists in preparing monthly financial and cost reports.
- Assists in posting information to general ledger.
- Assists in reconciling general ledger.
- Ensure compliance with current healthcare regulations, medical laws, federal and state laws, and high ethical standards.
- Processes all accounts payable invoices.
- Processes accounts payable checks and voided checks.

Education:

- High school diploma or GED and one year of customer service experience required, such as administrative, physician's office, appointment scheduler or retail/service industry.
- Associate degree and coursework in a healthcare related field is preferred (e.g., Administrative Clinic Assistant, Medical Office, Medical Assistant, Healthcare/Medical Receptionist or comparable).

Experience:

- Minimum two years of accounts payable experience, preferably in healthcare and exposure to general ledger accounting.

Competency requirements:

Knowledge:

- Knowledge of and experience with [vendor-specific EHR] is preferred.
- Knowledge of Electronic Health Systems
- Knowledge of Practice Management Systems
- Knowledge of proper phone etiquette and phone handling skills.
- Knowledge of organizational policies, procedures, and systems.
- Knowledge of office management techniques and practices.
- Knowledge of computer systems, programs, and applications.
- Knowledge of research methods and procedures sufficient to compile data and prepare reports.
- Knowledge of grammar, spelling, and punctuation.
- General knowledge of healthcare terminology preferred.
- Knowledge of purchasing, budgeting, and inventory control.

Skills:

- Skill in taking and transcribing dictation and in the operation of office equipment.
- This position requires strong working knowledge of managed care plans, insurance carriers, referrals and precertification procedures.
- Ability to communicate in English, both verbally and in writing.
- Additional languages preferred.
- CPT and ICD-10 coding abilities preferred.
- Must possess strong human relations, communication, problem solving, and organizational skills to interact with a variety of customers and personnel, both within and outside the institution.

- Must be able to work independently and in a team environment.
- Requires strong personal computer skills, communication skills, problem solving, continuous improvement and teaming skills.
- Maintains a broad knowledge of clinical, financial, and administrative systems/applications and processes.
- Serves as a resource on department and institutional initiatives; shares knowledge with customers and colleagues.
- Demonstrated verbal and written communication skills.

Abilities:

- Must maintain regular and acceptable attendance; may be required to work weekend, holiday or OT hours.
- Ability to establish and maintain effective working relationships with other employees and the public.
- Ability to work under pressure, communicate and present information.
- Ability to read, interpret, and apply clinic policies and procedures.
- Ability to identify problems, recommend solutions, organize and analyze information.
- Ability to establish priorities and coordinate work activities.
- Exposure to electronic health record preferred.
- Ability to work independently, be goal-directed and have strong organizational skills.
- Effectively multitask without compromising quality.
- Ability to comprehend and excel in both verbal and written communication, including proper telephone etiquette, face-to-face interactions, and electronic communications.
- Ability to communicate with individuals and small groups with credibility and confidence.
- Ability to handle difficult situations, remain calm under stress, manage emotional situations, display empathy

and maintain positive communication during a rapidly changing/dynamic environment.

- Turn problems into opportunities by developing innovative and creative solutions.
- Demonstrate a friendly, positive attitude, display energy and drive in performing daily responsibilities.
- Must be flexible as well as easily adapt to a changing work environment which will require ongoing maintenance of job-related skills/activities.
- Must be willing to adjust work schedules in response to department or clinical needs.
- Able to manage and prioritize tasks simultaneously while working directly with patients who may exhibit diverse needs.

Equipment Operated:

- Standard office equipment including computers, fax machines, copiers, printers, telephones, etc.

Work Environment:

Position is in a well-lit office environment. Occasional evening and weekend work.

Mental/Physical Requirements:

- Involves sitting approximately 90 percent of the day, walking or standing the remainder.
- Combination of sitting, standing, bending, light lifting and walking.
- Requires a full range of body motion including manual and finger dexterity and hand-eye coordination.
- Requires corrected vision and hearing to a normal range.
- Requires the ability to manage stressful situations.
- Occasional stress from varying demands.
- Requires corrected vision and hearing to a normal range.
- Requires the ability to manage stressful situations.
- Occasional stress from varying demands.

Disclaimer: This description is intended to provide only basic guidelines for meeting job requirements. Responsibilities, knowledge, skills, abilities, and working conditions may change as needs of the organization evolve and on an organization by organization basis.

Job Title: Accounting Manager

Department: Administration
Immediate Supervisor Title: Practice Administrator
Job Supervisory Responsibilities: Designated individuals in the accounting department

General Summary:

A professional position responsible for assisting in determining financial objectives; analyzing and reporting accounting variances; developing and monitoring accounting reports and control mechanisms.

Essential Job Responsibilities:

- Directs and coordinates activities of accounting staff including payroll, accounts payable, general ledger, tax payments, fixes assets, and purchasing activities.
- Develops, implements, and maintains accounting policies and procedures regarding patient accounts and reimbursements by patient, insurance, and other third-party reimbursors.
- Ensure compliance with current healthcare regulations, medical laws, federal and state laws, and high ethical standards.
- Closes the monthly financial records according to generally accepted accounting principles, which include preparing journal entries, reconciling accounting, and functioning as the primary accountant.
- Oversees operating budgets and ensures expenditures do not exceed budgetary limits.
- Prepares for and assists in the annual independent audit of the organization by the accounting firm.

Education:

- Bachelor's degree in accounting or finance.

- Individuals may also need to complete additional coursework upon hire.
- Completion of a medical terminology course or successful completion within six months of employment.

Experience:

- Minimum four years of experience in accounting management, including two years in a healthcare organization.

Other Requirements:

- Must be available to have a mixed schedule of opening and closing the office and the ability to be flexible with schedule when needed.
- MGMA certification.
- CPA preferred.

Competency Requirements:

Knowledge:

- Knowledge of and experience with [vendor-specific EHR] is preferred.
- Knowledge of Electronic Health Systems in any case
- Knowledge of Practice Management Systems
- Knowledge of proper phone etiquette and phone handling skills.
- Knowledge of organizational policies, procedures, and systems.
- Knowledge of office management techniques and practices.
- Knowledge of computer systems, programs, and applications.
- Knowledge of grammar, spelling, and punctuation.
- General knowledge of healthcare terminology preferred.
- Knowledge of purchasing, budgeting, and inventory control.

- Knowledge of advanced financial accounting, analysis, and reporting to design, modify, and manage an accounting system.
- Knowledge of automated accounting systems and governmental regulations.
- Knowledge of reimbursement procedures to compile and allocate cost information to specific accounts.

Skills:

- Skill in taking and transcribing dictation and in the operation of office equipment.
- This position requires strong working knowledge of managed care plans, insurance carriers, referrals and precertification procedures.
- Ability to communicate in English, both verbally and in writing.
- Additional languages preferred.
- CPT and ICD-10 coding abilities preferred.
- Must possess strong human relations, communication, problem solving, and organizational skills to interact with a variety of customers and personnel, both within and outside the institution.
- Must be able to work independently and in a team environment.
- Requires strong personal computer skills, communication skills, problem solving, continuous improvement and teaming skills.
- Maintains a broad knowledge of clinical, financial, and administrative systems/applications and processes.
- Serves as a resource on department and institutional initiatives; shares knowledge with customers and colleagues.
- Demonstrated verbal and written communication skills.
- Skill in budgeting, preparing financial reports, and computer applications.
- Skill in exercising initiative, judgment, discretion, and decision-making to achieve organizational objectives.

- Skill in identifying and resolving accounting problems.

Abilities:

- Must maintain regular and acceptable attendance; may be required to work weekend, holiday or OT hours.
- Ability to establish and maintain effective working relationships with other employees and the public.
- Ability to work under pressure, communicate and present information.
- Ability to read, interpret, and apply clinic policies and procedures.
- Ability to identify problems, recommend solutions, organize and analyze information.
- Ability to establish priorities and coordinate work activities.
- Ability to work independently, be goal-directed and have strong organizational skills.
- Effectively multitask without compromising quality.
- Ability to comprehend and excel in both verbal and written communication, including proper telephone etiquette, face-to-face interactions, and electronic communications.
- Ability to communicate with individuals and small groups with credibility and confidence.
- Ability to handle difficult situations, remain calm under stress, manage emotional situations, display empathy and maintain positive communication during a rapidly changing/dynamic environment.
- Turn problems into opportunities by developing innovative and creative solutions.
- Demonstrate a friendly, positive attitude, display energy and drive in performing daily responsibilities.
- Must be flexible as well as easily adapt to a changing work environment which will require ongoing maintenance of job-related skills/activities.
- Must be willing to adjust work schedules in response to department or clinical needs.

- Able to manage and prioritize tasks simultaneously while working directly with patients who may exhibit diverse needs. Ability to delegate responsibility and authority to staff.
- Ability to work creatively with management and department staff to achieve objectives.
- Ability to communicate effectively with all levels of management regarding financial policies.

Equipment Operated:

- Standard office equipment including computers, fax machines, copiers, printers, telephones, etc.

Work Environment:

Position is in a well-lit office environment. Occasional evening and weekend work.

Mental/Physical Requirements:

- Involves sitting approximately 90 percent of the day, walking or standing the remainder.
- Combination of sitting, standing, bending, light lifting and walking.
- Requires a full range of body motion including manual and finger dexterity and hand-eye coordination.
- Requires corrected vision and hearing to a normal range.
- Requires the ability to manage stressful situations.
- Occasional stress from varying demands.

Disclaimer: This description is intended to provide only basic guidelines for meeting job requirements. Responsibilities, knowledge, skills, abilities, and working conditions may change as needs of the organization evolve and on an organization by organization basis.

Job Title: Controller

Department: Financial Management
Immediate Supervisor Title: : Chief Financial Officer
Job Supervisory Responsibilities: Financial
Management department staff

General Summary:

A professional position responsible for organizing and maintaining financial accounting systems, including accounts payable, general ledger, accounts receivable, employee payroll, cash disbursements, financial statements, and tax information.

Essential Job Responsibilities:

- Develops and plans department objectives with chief financial officer and staff including short- and long-range accounting programs in budgeting, profit analysis, accounting systems, Medicare cost reporting, and internal auditing.
- Directs financial accounting functions to ensure timely and accurate reporting of financial information.
- Develops and implements policies and procedures to ensure compliance with regulatory agencies.
- Works with finance director to develop and approve financial statements, including balance sheets, profit/loss statements, and analysis of variances in accounts, ratios, income/expense, as well as investment analysis, e.g., effects of fee changes on costs and profits, return on investment.
- Reviews all third-party contracts and monitors contract revenues.
- Interacts with auditors, lenders, and other third-party agencies regarding accounting functions.

- Ensure compliance with current healthcare regulations, medical laws, federal and state laws, and high ethical standards.
- Develops and monitors the internal audit program to ensure internal financial controls. Oversees the annual financial audit and any other special audits.
- Directs the preparation of statistical information and reports for management, government, and other agencies.

Education:

- Bachelor's degree in finance or accounting.

Experience:

- Minimum three years of financial management experience, including two years in a healthcare organization.

Other Requirements:

- CPA preferred.

Competency requirements:

Knowledge:

- Knowledge of finance and accounting functions, including budgeting, credit, investments, and internal controls.
- Knowledge of computer systems, spreadsheet and financial systems programs and applications.
- Knowledge of management practices to lead assigned staff.
- Knowledge of strategic business objectives and employee performance objectives.

Skills:

- Skill in analyzing financial data and preparing appropriate related reports.

- Skill in relating organizational objectives to financial policies on costs, fees, credit, etc.
- Skill in exercising initiative, judgment, discretion, and decision-making to achieve organizational objectives.
- Skill in establishing and maintaining effective working relationships with patients, medical staff, auditors, and the public.
- Skill in identifying and resolving accounting and financial problems.

Abilities:

- Ability to delegate responsibility and authority to staff and work under multiple priorities.
- Ability to work creatively with management and department staff to achieve objectives.
- Ability to communicate effectively and clearly.

Equipment Operated:

- Standard office equipment including computers, fax machines, copiers, printers, telephones, etc.

Work Environment:

Position is in a well-lit office environment. Occasional evening and weekend work.

Mental/Physical Requirements:

- Involves sitting approximately 90 percent of the day, walking or standing the remainder.
- Combination of sitting, standing, bending, light lifting and walking.
- Requires a full range of body motion including manual and finger dexterity and hand-eye coordination.
- Requires corrected vision and hearing to a normal range.
- Requires the ability to manage stressful situations.
- Occasional stress from varying demands.

Disclaimer: This description is intended to provide only basic guidelines for meeting job requirements. Responsibilities, knowledge, skills, abilities, and working conditions may change as needs of the organization evolve and on an organization by organization basis.

Job Title: Chief Financial Officer

Department: Administration
Immediate Supervisor Title: Board of Directors
Job Supervisory Responsibilities: Controller, accounting manager, senior accountant, and business office manager; indirect supervision of all members of the Billing/accounting department.

General Summary:

An executive position responsible for directing the organization's financial planning and accounting practices as well as its relationship with lending institutions, pay sources, and the financial community.

Essential Job Responsibilities:

- Interacts with clinic management staff in developing the strategic plan and its financial planning component.
- Oversees and directs budgeting, audit, tax, accounting, purchasing, long-range forecasting, and insurance activities for the organization.
- Evaluates the organization's financial position and issues periodic reports on the organization's financial stability, liquidity, and growth.
- Develops and implements financial policies and procedures and ensures compliance.
- Assures implementation of internal controls and generally accepted accounting principles accounting.
- Ensure compliance with current healthcare regulations, medical laws, federal and state laws, and high ethical standards.
- Supervises the analysis of costs and makes rate recommendations to ensure appropriate income/cash flow.
- Oversees and directs the preparation and issuance of the organization's annual tax and other reports.

- Prepares or reviews financial statements for Board of Directors.

Education:

- Master's degree in business administration, accounting, or finance.

Experience:

- Eight to ten years of experience in financial/accounting management experience in healthcare financial management strongly preferred.

Other Requirements:

- CPA required.
- MGMA certification.

Competency requirements:

Knowledge:

- Knowledge of the principles of financial management sufficient to direct professional staff and coordinate all aspects involved with fiscal requirements.
- Knowledge of clinic financial and budgetary practices to develop annual budget, analyze financial data and patterns, and prepare financial statements.
- Knowledge of clinic's strategic business objectives and employee performance objectives.
- Knowledge of governmental and healthcare fiscal regulations and reporting requirements.

Skills:

- Skill in exercising a high degree of initiative, judgment, discretion, and decision-making to achieve objectives.
- Skill in evaluating operations as they relate to policies, goals and objectives, costs, and rate levels.
- Skill in establishing and maintaining effective working relationships with patients, medical staff, and the public.

- Skill in identifying and resolving accounting and financial problems.

Abilities:

- Ability to create an atmosphere that encourages motivation, innovation, and high performance.
- Ability to delegate responsibility and authority to staff.
- Ability to communicate effectively and clearly.

Equipment Operated:

- Standard office equipment including computers, fax machines, copiers, printers, telephones, etc.

Work Environment:

Position is in a well-lit office environment. Occasional evening and weekend work.

Mental/Physical Requirements:

- Involves sitting approximately 90 percent of the day, walking or standing the remainder.
- Combination of sitting, standing, bending, light lifting and walking.
- Requires a full range of body motion including manual and finger dexterity and hand-eye coordination.
- Requires corrected vision and hearing to a normal range.
- Requires the ability to manage stressful situations.
- Occasional stress from varying demands.

Disclaimer: This description is intended to provide only basic guidelines for meeting job requirements. Responsibilities, knowledge, skills, abilities, and working conditions may change as needs of the organization evolve and on an organization by organization basis.

Job Title: Credit Manager

Department: Financial Management
Immediate Supervisor Title: : Chief Financial Officer
Job Supervisory Responsibilities: Medical Billing/Coding Specialist

General Summary:

- A management position responsible for ensuring currency of accounts receivable including monitoring for delinquent payments.

Essential Job Responsibilities:

- Gathers data on daily, monthly, and yearly basis to determine credit status of clinic patient accounts.
- Monitors private-pay patient accounts for delinquent payments and determines course of action.
- Follows clinic collection policy guidelines and refers to collection agency upon physician approval.
- Ensure compliance with current healthcare regulations, medical laws, federal and state laws, and high ethical standards.
- Uses collection management reports to keep accounts receivable current.
- Runs routine insurance claim forms and statements to check on credit status.
- Assists with filing claims in cases of bankruptcy or to estates of deceased patients for unpaid accounts.

Education:

- Bachelor's degree in business administration or related field.

Experience:

- Minimum three years of collection and management experience in a healthcare organization.

Other Requirements:

- Must be available to have a mixed schedule of opening and closing the office and the ability to be flexible with schedule when needed.
- MGMA certification.

Competency requirements:

Knowledge:

- Knowledge of collection methods, policies, and procedures.
- Knowledge of calculations to compute fees and interest.

Skills:

- Skill in using computer programs, spreadsheets, and applications for credit
- entry, retrieval, and modification.
- Skill in supervising staff and serving as resource to management.

Abilities:

- Ability to understand and interpret credit policies and regulations.
- Ability to respond to patients on credit matters in courteous fashion.
- Ability to examine medical documents for accuracy and completeness.
- Ability to communicate effectively and clearly.

Equipment Operated:

- Standard office equipment including computers, fax machines, copiers, printers, telephones, etc.

Work Environment:

Position is in a well-lit office environment. Occasional evening and weekend work.

Mental/Physical Requirements:

- Involves sitting approximately 90 percent of the day, walking or standing the remainder.
- Combination of sitting, standing, bending, light lifting and walking.
- Requires a full range of body motion including manual and finger dexterity and hand-eye coordination.
- Requires corrected vision and hearing to a normal range.
- Requires the ability to manage stressful situations.
- Occasional stress from varying demands.

Disclaimer: This description is intended to provide only basic guidelines for meeting job requirements. Responsibilities, knowledge, skills, abilities, and working conditions may change as needs of the organization evolve and on an organization by organization basis.

Job Title: Payroll Administrator

Department: Financial Management
Immediate Supervisor Title: Controller
Job Supervisory Responsibilities: Payroll Clerk

General Summary:

A position responsible for overseeing the payroll function for the organization.

Essential Job Responsibilities:

- Establishes systems and procedures that ensure the appropriate and timely payment of employees.
- Manages the preparation, distribution, and reporting processes for payroll.
- Oversees the calculation of wages, overtime, and deductions to ensure compliance with federal, state, and local laws and regulations.
- Generates reports from databases to disseminate information to internal departments and external entities.
- Enhance patient experiences; optimizing company reputation.
- Ensure compliance with current healthcare regulations, medical laws, federal and state laws, and high ethical standards.
- Performs reconciliations of payroll information and accounting information for budgetary purposes.

Education:

- College degree preferred with accounting and finance courses.

Experience:

- Minimum five years of experience as a payroll administrator.

Other Requirements:

- Must be available to have a mixed schedule of opening and closing the office and the ability to be flexible with schedule when needed.

Competency requirements:

Knowledge:

- Knowledge of complex payroll practices and wage/hour laws, including tax filing and other financial responsibilities.
- Knowledge of state-of-the-art payroll programs and payroll systems.
- Understanding of the principles of accounting as they relate to payroll functions.

Skills:

- This position requires strong working knowledge of managed care plans, insurance carriers, referrals and precertification procedures.
- Skill in exercising a high degree of initiative, judgment, and discretion.
- Skill in analyzing situations accurately and taking effective action.
- Skill in establishing and maintaining effective working relationships.
- Skill in organizing work, delegating and achieving goals and objectives.
- Skill in interpreting and analyzing payroll data.
- Effective communication skills, both verbal and written.
- Effective management skills.

Abilities:

- Ability to accurately perform mathematical functions and statistical analysis.
- Ability to prepare and analyze comprehensive reports.
- Ability to maintain confidentiality of financial matters.
- Ability to work effectively with others.
- Ability to ensure compliance with deadlines.

Equipment Operated:

- Standard office equipment, including computers, fax machines, copiers, printers, telephones, etc.

Work Environment:

Position is in a well-lit office environment. Occasional evening and weekend work.

Mental/Physical Requirements:

- Involves sitting approximately 90 percent of the day, walking or standing the remainder.
- Combination of sitting, standing, bending, light lifting and walking.
- Requires a full range of body motion including manual and finger dexterity and hand-eye coordination.
- Lifting up to 20 pounds.
- Requires corrected vision and hearing to a normal range.
- Requires the ability to manage stressful situations.
- Occasional stress from varying demands.

Disclaimer: This description is intended to provide only basic guidelines for meeting job requirements. Responsibilities, knowledge, skills, abilities, and working conditions may change as needs of the organization evolve and on an organization by organization basis.

Job Title: Payroll Clerk

Department: Financial Management

Immediate Supervisor Title: Controller

Job Supervisory Responsibilities:

General Summary:

A position responsible for preparation of payroll.

Essential Job Responsibilities:

- Processes employee time sheets and checks for accuracy.
- Clarifies inconsistencies with supervisors.
- Verifies sick leave, vacation hours, and overtime by comparing authorization forms to time reports.
- Enhance patient experiences; optimizing company reputation.
- Ensure compliance with current healthcare regulations, medical laws, federal and state laws, and high ethical standards.
- Processes COBRA, jury duty, short- and long-term disability payments.
- Adds and deletes employees from payroll and accounting systems.
- Processes employment verifications forms, wage assignments, levies, and child support.
- Distributes payroll checks to the appropriate department.

Education:

- High school diploma; some college preferred.

Experience:

- Minimum two years of payroll experience.

Other Requirements:

- Must be available to have a mixed schedule of opening and closing the office and the ability to be flexible with schedule when needed.

Competency Requirements:

Knowledge:

- Understanding of payroll practices as well as federal and state wage/hour laws.
- Understanding of various payroll systems.

Skills:

- Must be able to multi-task and have attention to detail.
- Perform accurate data entry, both alpha and numeric.

Abilities:

- Ability to work efficiently and accurately within specific deadlines.
- Ability to work with and learn new systems that are implemented.
- Ability to prepare comprehensive reports.
- Ability to effectively communicate and work with other people.

Equipment Operated:

- Standard office equipment including computers, fax machines, copiers, printers, telephones, etc.

Work Environment:

Position is in a well-lit office environment.
Occasional evening and weekend work.

Mental/Physical Requirements:

- Involves sitting approximately 90 % of the day, walking or standing the remainder.

- Combination of sitting, standing, bending, light lifting and walking.
- Requires a full range of body motion including manual and finger dexterity and hand-eye coordination.
- Lifting up to 20 pounds.
- Requires corrected vision and hearing to a normal range.
- Requires the ability to manage stressful situations.
- Occasional stress from varying demands.

Disclaimer: This description is intended to provide only basic guidelines for meeting job requirements. Responsibilities, knowledge, skills, abilities, and working conditions may change as needs of the organization evolve and on an organization by organization basis.

Job Title: Senior Accountant

Department: Financial Management
Immediate Supervisor Title: Chief Financial Officer or Controller
Job Supervisory Responsibilities: Assigned accounting staff

General Summary:

A management position responsible for managing, maintaining, and analyzing accounting management information including general ledger activity through financial statements.

Essential Job Responsibilities:

- Prepares accurate monthly financial statements.
- Analyzes, reviews, and adjusts income and expense information as to adequacy, form, and source.
- Enhance patient experiences; optimizing company reputation.
- Ensure compliance with current healthcare regulations, medical laws, federal and state laws, and high ethical standards.
- Maintains general ledger, including preparing financial schedules and writing journal entries for such items as interest income, prepaid insurance, FICA payments, etc.
- Maintains cash schedules, inspects account status, transfers cash as necessary to cover disbursements.
- Conducts reconciliations of balance sheet asset and liability accounts to ensure correctness. Identifies and resolves discrepancies.
- Maintains amortization schedules for lease agreements, mortgages, bank notes, and bond premiums.

Education:

- Bachelor's degree in accounting.

Experience:

- Minimum three years of experience in professional accounting and management experience including one year in healthcare.

Other Requirements:

- Must be available to have a mixed schedule of opening and closing the office and the ability to be flexible with schedule when needed.
- MGMA certification.

Competency Requirements:

Knowledge:

- Knowledge of accounting practices to understand and interpret various accounting systems.
- Knowledge of budgeting and cost accounting principles.
- Knowledge of GAAP in their current form.

Skills:

- Skill in defining problems, collecting data, interpreting financial material.
- Skill in preparing statistical and narrative accounting and auditing reports.

Abilities:

- Ability to evaluate accounting systems.
- Ability to use cost accounting reports to recommend alternatives for controlling operations.
- Ability to perform mathematical computations and compute ratios and percentages.
- Ability to communicate clearly.

Equipment Operated:

- Standard office equipment including computers, fax machines, copiers, printers, telephones, etc.

Work Environment:

Position is in a well-lit office environment.
Occasional evening and weekend work.

Mental/Physical Requirements:

- Involves sitting approximately 90 % of the day, walking or standing the remainder.
- Combination of sitting, standing, bending, light lifting and walking.
- Requires a full range of body motion including manual and finger dexterity and hand-eye coordination.
- Lifting up to 20 pounds.
- Requires corrected vision and hearing to a normal range.
- Requires the ability to manage stressful situations.
- Occasional stress from varying demands.

Disclaimer: This description is intended to provide only basic guidelines for meeting job requirements. Responsibilities, knowledge, skills, abilities, and working conditions may change as needs of the organization evolve and on an organization by organization basis.

Job Title: Staff Accountant

Department: Financial Management
Immediate Supervisor Title: Accounting Manager
Job Supervisory Responsibilities: None

General Summary:

A position responsible for assisting accounting manager with accounting functions including reporting of financial operations.

Essential Job Responsibilities:

- Prepares monthly general and standard journal entries, financial statements and comparative reports, account reconciliations, cost reports.
- Assists independent auditors with interim and year-end audits and verifies accuracy of reports.
- Prepares federal, state, and other governmental reports such as annual tax returns and ERISA reports.
- Maintains and reviews cost center and appropriation accounts, including trial balances, to verify accuracy with coding, classifying, and posting.
- Prepares reports of budget expenditures, revenues, and account or fund balances.
- Supervises payroll activities and resolves payroll problems.
- Ensure compliance with current healthcare regulations, medical laws, federal and state laws, and high ethical standards.

Education:

- Bachelor's degree in business administration, preferably in accounting.

Experience:

- Minimum three years of accounting experience, including one year of accounting experience specifically in healthcare.

Other Requirements:

- Must be available to have a mixed schedule of opening and closing the office and the ability to be flexible with schedule when needed.
- MGMA certification.

Competency Requirements:

Knowledge:

- Knowledge of the generally accepted accounting principles.(GAAP)
- Knowledge of budgeting and cost accounting principles.

Skills:

- Excellent analytical and math skills.
- Good communication skills.
- Skill in dealing with multiple projects and interruptions.
- Strong organizational skills; attention to detail.
- Ability to communicate in English, both verbally and in writing.
- Additional languages preferred.

Abilities:

- Ability to analyze financial reports.
- Ability to prepare accounting reports.
- Ability to work independently and meet deadlines as assigned.
- Ability to maintain effective working relationships.
- Ability to communicate with individuals and small groups with credibility and confidence.
- Ability to handle difficult situations, remain calm under stress, manage emotional situations, display empathy

and maintain positive communication during a rapidly changing/dynamic environment.

- Turn problems into opportunities by developing innovative and creative solutions.
- Demonstrate a friendly, positive attitude, display energy and drive in performing daily responsibilities.
- Must be flexible as well as easily adapt to a changing work environment which will require ongoing maintenance of job-related skills/activities.

Equipment Operated:

- Standard office equipment including computers, fax machines, copiers, printers, telephones, etc.

Work Environment:

Position is in a well-lit office environment.
Occasional evening and weekend work.

Mental/Physical Requirements:

- Involves sitting approximately 90 % of the day, walking or standing the remainder.
- Combination of sitting, standing, bending, light lifting and walking.
- Requires a full range of body motion including manual and finger dexterity and hand-eye coordination.
- Lifting up to 20 pounds.
- Requires corrected vision and hearing to a normal range.
- Requires the ability to manage stressful situations.
- Occasional stress from varying demands.

Disclaimer: This description is intended to provide only basic guidelines for meeting job requirements. Responsibilities, knowledge, skills, abilities, and working conditions may change as needs of the organization evolve and on an organization by organization basis.

Job Title: Benefits Specialist

Department: Human Resources
Immediate Supervisor Title: Human Resources Manager
Job Supervisory Responsibilities:

General Summary:

An administrative position responsible for coordinating and administrating all employee benefits programs.

Essential Job Responsibilities:

- Coordinates and administers health, dental, and life insurance plans; disability; flexible spending accounts; retirement savings plan; profit sharing programs; tuition reimbursement; COBRA; Legal Plans; Wellness plans: and personal leaves of absence.
- Review for accuracy and maintains the human resources database.
- Creates reports regarding benefits.
- Develops and conducts new employee orientation session for new hires to explain benefit packages available.
- Ensures compliance with medical practice policies and procedures and federal, state, and local laws and regulations.

Education:

- Bachelor's degree in business administration or health-related field
- Basic Life Support (BLS) may be required in some areas.
- Individuals may also need to complete additional coursework upon hire.
- Completion of a medical terminology course or successful completion within six months of employment.

Experience:

- Minimum three years of experience in human resources in a healthcare setting, preferably with experience in benefits.

Other Requirements:

- Must be available to have a mixed schedule of opening and closing the office and the ability to be flexible with schedule when needed.

Competency requirements:

Knowledge:

- Knowledge of and experience with [vendor-specific EHR] is preferred.
- Knowledge of Electronic Health Systems in any case
- Knowledge of Practice Management Systems
- Knowledge of proper phone etiquette and phone handling skills.
- Knowledge of organizational policies, procedures, and systems.
- Knowledge of office management techniques and practices.
- Knowledge of computer systems, programs, and applications.
- Knowledge of research methods and procedures sufficient to compile data and prepare reports.
- Knowledge of grammar, spelling, and punctuation.
- General knowledge of healthcare terminology preferred.
- Knowledge of purchasing, budgeting, and inventory control.

Skills:

- Skill in taking and transcribing dictation and in the operation of office equipment.

- This position requires strong working knowledge of managed care plans, insurance carriers, referrals and precertification procedures.
- Ability to communicate in English, both verbally and in writing.
- Additional languages preferred.
- CPT and ICD-10 coding abilities preferred.
- Must possess strong human relations, communication, problem solving, and organizational skills to interact with a variety of customers and personnel, both within and outside the institution.
- Must be able to work independently and in a team environment.
- Requires strong personal computer skills, communication skills, problem solving, continuous improvement and teaming skills.
- Maintains a broad knowledge of clinical, financial, and administrative systems/applications and processes.
- Serves as a resource on department and institutional initiatives; shares knowledge with customers and colleagues.
- Demonstrated verbal and written communication skills.

Abilities:

- Must maintain regular and acceptable attendance; may be required to work weekend, holiday or OT hours.
- Ability to establish and maintain effective working relationships with other employees and the public.
- Ability to work under pressure, communicate and present information.
- Ability to read, interpret, and apply clinic policies and procedures.
- Ability to identify problems, recommend solutions, organize and analyze information.
- Ability to establish priorities and coordinate work activities.
- Exposure to electronic health record preferred.

- Ability to work independently, be goal-directed and have strong organizational skills.
- Effectively multitask without compromising quality.
- Ability to comprehend and excel in both verbal and written communication, including proper telephone etiquette, face-to-face interactions, and electronic communications.
- Ability to communicate with individuals and small groups with credibility and confidence.
- Ability to handle difficult situations, remain calm under stress, manage emotional situations, display empathy and maintain positive communication during a rapidly changing/dynamic environment.
- Turn problems into opportunities by developing innovative and creative solutions.
- Demonstrate a friendly, positive attitude, display energy and drive in performing daily responsibilities.
- Must be flexible as well as easily adapt to a changing work environment which will require ongoing maintenance of job-related skills/activities.
- Must be willing to adjust work schedules in response to department or clinical needs.
- Able to manage and prioritize tasks simultaneously while working directly with patients who may exhibit diverse needs.

Equipment Operated:

- Standard office equipment including computers, fax machines, copiers, printers, telephones, etc.

Work Environment:

Position is in a well-lit office environment. Occasional evening and weekend work.

Mental/Physical Requirements:

- Involves sitting approximately 90 percent of the day, walking or standing the remainder.
- Combination of sitting, standing, bending, light lifting and walking.
- Requires a full range of body motion including manual and finger dexterity and hand-eye coordination.
- Requires corrected vision and hearing to a normal range.
- Requires the ability to manage stressful situations.
- Occasional stress from varying demands.

Disclaimer: This description is intended to provide only basic guidelines for meeting job requirements. Responsibilities, knowledge, skills, abilities, and working conditions may change as needs of the organization evolve and on an organization by organization basis.

Job Title: Compensation Specialist

Department: Human Resources
Immediate Supervisor Title: Human Resources Director
Job Supervisory Responsibilities:

General Summary:

A clerical position responsible for coordinating the compensation program.

Essential Job Responsibilities:

- Manages and maintains the payroll system.
- Facilitates promotion/transfer functions related to salaries.
- Analyzes current healthcare compensation trends and recommends changes as needed.
- Maintains compliance with federal, state, and local employment laws and regulations.
- Maintains all staff and personnel files.
- Enhance patient experiences; optimizing company reputation.
- Ensure compliance with current healthcare regulations, medical laws, federal and state laws, and high ethical standards.

Education:

- Bachelor's degree, preferably in business.
- Individuals may also need to complete additional coursework upon hire.
- Completion of a medical terminology course or successful completion within six months of employment.

Experience:

- Minimum two years of experience in human resources, preferably in a healthcare setting. Compensation background desirable.

Other Requirements:

- Must be available to have a mixed schedule of opening and closing the office and the ability to be flexible with schedule when needed.
- MGMA certification.

Competency requirements:

Knowledge:

- Knowledge of policies and procedures to manage operations and ensure effective patient care.
- Knowledge of the principles and practices of healthcare administration, fiscal management, and government regulations and reimbursements.
- Knowledge of current compensation and administration requirements.
- Knowledge of federal, state, and local regulations related to compensation and employment laws.
- Knowledge of payroll systems.

Skills:

- Skill in using compensation and payroll systems.
- Skill in understanding employment law by accurate recording and reports in compliance with regulations.
- Skill in exercising a high degree of initiative, judgment, and discretion.
- Skill in analyzing situations accurately and taking effective action.
- Skill in establishing and maintaining effective working relationships.
- Skill in organizing work, delegating and achieving goals and objectives.

- Skill in exercising judgment and discretion in developing, interpreting, and implementing departmental policies and procedures.

Abilities:

- Must maintain regular and acceptable attendance; may be required to work weekend, holiday or OT hours.
- Ability to establish and maintain effective working relationships with other employees and the public.
- Ability to work under pressure, communicate and present information.
- Ability to read, interpret, and apply clinic policies and procedures.
- Ability to identify problems, recommend solutions, organize and analyze information.
- Ability to establish priorities and coordinate work activities.
- Ability to work effectively with all levels of personnel including physicians, managers, and other staff.
- Ability to be highly efficient, organized, and accurate in work.

Equipment Operated:

- Standard office equipment including computers, fax machines, copiers, printers, telephones, etc.

Work Environment:

Position is in a well-lit office environment.
Occasional evening and weekend work.

Mental/Physical Requirements:

- Involves sitting approximately 90 percent of the day, walking or standing the remainder.
- Combination of sitting, standing, bending, light lifting and walking.

- Requires a full range of body motion including manual and finger dexterity and hand-eye coordination.
- Lifting up to 20 pounds.
- Requires corrected vision and hearing to a normal range.
- Requires the ability to manage stressful situations.
- Occasional stress from varying demands.

Disclaimer: This description is intended to provide only basic guidelines for meeting job requirements. Responsibilities, knowledge, skills, abilities, and working conditions may change as needs of the organization evolve and on an organization by organization basis.

Job Title: Human Resources Assistant

Department: Human Resources
Immediate Supervisor Title: Human Resources Director
Job Supervisory Responsibilities: None

General Summary:

A clerical position responsible for functions related to payroll, personnel information, and employee documentation.

Essential Job Responsibilities:

- Ensures new employees receive appropriate items including security card, time card, insurance/benefit information, orientation materials.
- Creates photo ID.
- Adds data to employee census.
- Gives preliminary recommendations for new employee benefits.
- Ensures terminated employee data are removed from appropriate employee databases, including insurance/ benefits, time/leave data, employee census, and file is moved to inactive status.
- Maintains employee address and phone extension lists and emergency contact information.
- Coordinates special events including employee birthdays, holiday get-togethers, and other special events.
- Participates in annual open enrollment benefit period and processes benefit documents.

Education:

- High school diploma or GED and one year of customer service experience required, such as administrative, physician's office, appointment scheduler or retail/ service industry.

- Some college preferred.

Experience:

- Minimum two years of experience in administrative assistant position, preferably in healthcare.

Other Requirements:

- Must be available to have a mixed schedule of opening and closing the office and the ability to be flexible with schedule when needed.

Competency requirements:

Knowledge:

- Knowledge of payroll and employment documentation.
- Knowledge of how to use computers and human resources software applications.
- Knowledge of employee benefits.

Skills:

- Skill in using human resources computer capabilities including database management software.
- Skill in clear presentation of benefits information.

Abilities:

- Ability to establish/maintain effective relationships with staff at all levels.
- Ability to handle sensitive and confidential employee information in a professional manner.
- Ability to plan and coordinate multiple administrative projects.

Equipment Operated:

- Standard office equipment including computers, fax machines, copiers, printers, telephones, etc.

Work Environment:

Position is in a well-lit office environment.
Occasional evening and weekend work.

Mental/Physical Requirements:

- Lifting -- Not to exceed 50 lbs.
- Writing, Sitting, Bending, Visual acuity, Reading, Field of vision/peripheral
- Standing -- spends majority of the shift working sitting.
- Regularly required to use hands to finger, handle, or feel objects, tools, or controls; bend, reach with hands and arms; stoop, kneel, and talk and/or hear.
- Exposure to: Noise, Chemical vapors, Infectious Materials
- Combination of sitting, standing, bending, light lifting and walking.
- Requires a full range of body motion including manual and finger dexterity and hand-eye coordination.
- Requires corrected vision and hearing to a normal range.
- Requires the ability to manage stressful situations.
- Occasional stress from varying demands.

Disclaimer: This description is intended to provide only basic guidelines for meeting job requirements. Responsibilities, knowledge, skills, abilities, and working conditions may change as needs of the organization evolve and on an organization by organization basis.

Job Title: Human Resources Director

Department: Human Resources

Immediate Supervisor Title: Chief Executive Officer or Administrator

Job Supervisory Responsibilities: Human Resources Manager, Human Resources Assistant, Compensation Specialist, Recruiting Specialist, Benefits Specialist, Training Specialist

General Summary:

A management position responsible for directing and coordinating the policies and practices of human resources including staffing, compensation, benefits administration, and EEOC.

Essential Job Responsibilities:

- Ensures the development of departmental plans, goals, mission, policies/ procedures, budget. Ensures selection, training, monitoring, and evaluation of departmental staff.
- Develops/implements human resources plan for clinic including recruitment, selection, promotion/transfer, orientation, compensation administration, and labor relations in collaboration with management team.
- Educates/advises administrative and clinical managers on personnel issues including termination, labor disputes, morale.
- Oversees the conduct of compensation surveys and recommends changes to ensure clinic remains competitive with market rates for wages/salaries and benefits.
- Maintains/monitors records of worker's compensation, EEO, ADA, FMLA, unemployment, and other employee claims.
- Reviews exit interview data.

- Recommends changes to policy and training to ensure compliance with laws and regulations.
- Practices open-door policy to encourage employees to discuss grievances.
- Facilitates and mediates peer-to-peer and employee to supervisor discussion.
- Recommends and facilitates employee recognition efforts and events.
- Ensures employee assistance is available for emergency relief.

Education:

- Bachelor's degree in business administration or human resources. MBA is preferred.

Experience:

- Minimum seven years of experience in personnel management with progressively increasing level of responsibility. Minimum two years in the healthcare industry.

Other Requirements:

- Must be available to have a mixed schedule of opening and closing the office and the ability to be flexible with schedule when needed.
- SHRM certification.

Competency requirements:

Knowledge:

- Knowledge of organizational policies, procedures, and systems.
- Knowledge of office management techniques and practices.
- Knowledge of computer systems, programs, and applications.

- Knowledge of grammar, spelling, and punctuation.
- General knowledge of healthcare terminology preferred.
- Knowledge of federal and state employment/labor laws, clinic policies.
- Knowledge of how to conduct wage/salary and employee satisfaction surveys; to mediate personnel grievances/disputes; to analyze human resources data for critical indicators.
- Knowledge of compensation/benefits administration.

Skills:

- Ability to communicate in English, both verbally and in writing.
- Additional languages preferred.
- Must possess strong human relations, communication, problem solving, and organizational skills to interact with a variety of customers and personnel, both within and outside the institution.
- Must be able to work independently and in a team environment.
- Requires strong personal computer skills, communication skills, problem solving, continuous improvement and teaming skills.
- Maintains a broad knowledge of clinical, financial, and administrative systems/applications and processes.
- Serves as a resource on department and institutional initiatives; shares knowledge with customers and colleagues.
- Demonstrated verbal and written communication skills.
- Skill in staying abreast of the latest employment, labor, compensation, government regulations related to personnel.
- Skill in gathering/analyzing objective and subjective data on personnel matters and facilitation resolution.
- Skill in advising/educating managers on human resources best practices including employee training, motivation, development, discipline/ termination.

Abilities:

- Must maintain regular and acceptable attendance; may be required to work weekend, holiday or OT hours.
- Ability to establish and maintain effective working relationships with other employees and the public.
- Ability to work under pressure, communicate and present information.
- Ability to read, interpret, and apply clinic policies and procedures.
- Ability to identify problems, recommend solutions, organize and analyze information.
- Ability to establish priorities and coordinate work activities.
- Exposure to electronic health record preferred.
- Ability to work independently, be goal-directed and have strong organizational skills.
- Effectively multitask without compromising quality.
- Ability to comprehend and excel in both verbal and written communication, including proper telephone etiquette, face-to-face interactions, and electronic communications.
- Ability to communicate with individuals and small groups with credibility and confidence.
- Ability to handle difficult situations, remain calm under stress, manage emotional situations, display empathy and maintain positive communication during a rapidly changing/dynamic environment.
- Turn problems into opportunities by developing innovative and creative solutions.
- Demonstrate a friendly, positive attitude, display energy and drive in performing daily responsibilities.
- Must be flexible as well as easily adapt to a changing work environment which will require ongoing maintenance of job-related skills/activities.
- Must be willing to adjust work schedules in response to department or clinical needs.

- Able to manage and prioritize tasks simultaneously while working directly with patients who may exhibit diverse needs.
- Ability to role model effectively with many types of people at all levels including as an employee advocate, a manager counsel, and a physician resource.
- Ability to direct the best use of the human resources management information system in reporting statistics.
- Ability to communicate effectively in written and verbal form.

Equipment Operated:

- Standard office equipment including computers, fax machines, copiers, printers, telephones, etc.

Work Environment:

Position is in a well-lit office environment. Occasional evening and weekend work.

Mental/Physical Requirements:

- Involves sitting approximately 90 percent of the day, walking or standing the remainder.
- Combination of sitting, standing, bending, light lifting and walking.
- Requires a full range of body motion including manual and finger dexterity and hand-eye coordination.
- Requires corrected vision and hearing to a normal range.
- Requires the ability to manage stressful situations.
- Occasional stress from varying demands.

Disclaimer: This description is intended to provide only basic guidelines for meeting job requirements. Responsibilities, knowledge, skills, abilities, and working conditions may change as needs of the organization evolve and on an organization by organization basis.

Job Title: Human Resources Manager

Department: Human Resources
Immediate Supervisor Title: Chief Executive Officer or Administrator
Job Supervisory Responsibilities: Human Resources staff

General Summary:

A management position responsible for directing and coordinating the policies and practices of human resources including staffing, compensation, benefits administration, and EEOC.

Essential Job Responsibilities:

- Ensures the development of departmental plans, goals, mission, policies/ procedures, budget.
- Ensures selection, training, monitoring, and evaluation of departmental staff.
- Develops/implements human resources plan for clinic including recruitment, selection, promotion/transfer, orientation, compensation administration, and labor relations in collaboration with management team.
- Educates/advises administrative and clinical managers on personnel issues including termination, labor disputes, morale.
- Reviews possible new benefits.
- Oversees the conduct of compensation surveys and recommends changes to ensure clinic remains competitive with market rates for wages/salaries and benefits.
- Maintains/monitors records of worker's compensation, EEO, ADA, FMLA, unemployment, and other employee claims.
- Reviews exit interview data.

- Recommends changes to policy and training to ensure compliance with laws and regulations.
- Practices open-door policy to encourage employees to discuss grievances.
- Facilitates peer-to-peer and employee–manager discussion/mediations.
- Recommends and facilitates employee recognition efforts and events.
- Ensures employee assistance is available for emergency relief.

Education:

- Bachelor's degree in business administration or human resources.

Experience:

- Minimum seven years of experience in personnel management with progressively increasing level of responsibility.
- Minimum two years in the healthcare industry.

Other Requirements:

- Must be available to have a mixed schedule of opening and closing the office and the ability to be flexible with schedule when needed.
- SHRM certification.

Competency requirements:

Knowledge:

- Knowledge of federal and state employment/labor laws, clinic policies.
- Knowledge of how to conduct wage/salary and employee satisfaction surveys; to mediate personnel grievances/disputes; to analyze human resources data for critical indicators.

- Knowledge of compensation/benefits administration.

Skills:

- Skill in staying abreast of the latest employment, labor, compensation, government regulations related to personnel.
- Skill in gathering/analyzing objective and subjective data on personnel matters and facilitation resolution.
- Skill in advising/educating managers on human resources best practices including employee training, motivation, development, discipline/ termination.

Abilities:

- Ability to role model effectively with many types of people at all levels including as an employee advocate, a manager counsel, and a physician resource.
- Ability to direct the best use of the human resources management information system in reporting statistics.
- Ability to communicate effectively in written and verbal form.

Equipment Operated:

- Standard office equipment including computers, fax machines, copiers, printers, telephones, etc.

Work Environment:

Position is in a well-lit office environment.
Occasional evening and weekend work.

Mental/Physical Requirements:

- Involves sitting approximately 90 percent of the day, walking or standing the remainder.
- Combination of sitting, standing, bending, light lifting and walking.
- Requires a full range of body motion including manual and finger dexterity and hand-eye coordination.

- Lifting up to 20 pounds.
- Requires corrected vision and hearing to a normal range.
- Requires the ability to manage stressful situations.
- Occasional stress from varying demands.

Disclaimer: This description is intended to provide only basic guidelines for meeting job requirements. Responsibilities, knowledge, skills, abilities, and working conditions may change as needs of the organization evolve and on an organization by organization basis.

Job Title: Recruiting Specialist

Department: Human Resources
Immediate Supervisor Title: Human Resources Manager
Job Supervisory Responsibilities: None

General Summary:

A position responsible for developing and implementing the full cycle of recruitment from the initial point of contact with qualified candidates through hiring.

Essential Job Responsibilities:

- Assisting and coordinating the development of strategic physician recruitment plans.
- Performing initial interview and screening processes to determine candidates' suitability.
- Hiring Physicians for healthcare organizations.
- Researching and participating in conferences, job fairs, and Physician Recruitment opportunity events.
- Visiting Physician practices to manage your understanding of the clinical requirements for recruitment purposes.
- Coordinating recruitment activities with HR personnel.
- Monitoring and maintaining the recruitment budget.
- Developing and maintaining advertising for recruiting efforts.
- Maintaining and managing outstanding communication with Physician candidates.
- Works with department directors and managers to identify professional staff needs and to develop a strategic recruitment plan.
- Enhance patient experiences; optimizing company reputation.
- Ensure compliance with current healthcare regulations, medical laws, federal and state laws, and high ethical standards.

133

- Actively advertises job openings using multiple media types including internal job posting boards, the Internet, job fairs, university career centers, job placement firms, national and local newspapers, and networking.
- Responsible for reviewing applicants and screening potential candidates including initial screening interviews.
- Reviews and checks all candidate references.

Education:

- Bachelor's degree in business or related field.

Experience:

- Minimum two years of experience in recruitment, preferably in a healthcare environment.

Other Requirements:

- Must be available to have a mixed schedule of opening and closing the office and the ability to be flexible with schedule when needed.

Competency requirements:

Knowledge:

- Knowledge of employment laws.
- Knowledge of various recruitment methods.
- Knowledge of customer service techniques.

Skills:

- Skill in problem solving.
- Skill in developing and implementing recruitment materials.
- Excellent organizational skills.

Abilities:

- Ability to project positive and professional image.

- Ability to coordinate and prioritize multiple tasks, projects, and schedules.
- Ability to establish and develop effective working relationships.

Equipment Operated:

- Standard office equipment including computers, fax machines, copiers, printers, telephones, etc.

Work Environment:

Position is in a well-lit office environment.
Occasional evening and weekend work.

Mental/Physical Requirements:

- Involves sitting approximately 90 percent of the day, walking or standing the remainder.
- Combination of sitting, standing, bending, light lifting and walking.
- Requires a full range of body motion including manual and finger dexterity and hand-eye coordination.
- Lifting up to 20 pounds.
- Requires corrected vision and hearing to a normal range.
- Requires the ability to manage stressful situations.
- Occasional stress from varying demands.

Disclaimer: This description is intended to provide only basic guidelines for meeting job requirements. Responsibilities, knowledge, skills, abilities, and working conditions may change as needs of the organization evolve and on an organization by organization basis.

Job Title: Training Specialist

Department: Human Resources
Immediate Supervisor Title: Human Resources Manager
Job Supervisory Responsibilities: None

General Summary:

A non-clinical position responsible for the assessment of professional educational needs and for the development, implementation, and evaluation of all education and training programs.

Essential Job Responsibilities:

- Regularly assesses the training needs of staff using interviews, surveys, observation, audits, and quality improvement data and facilitates the development of departmental training goals.
- Consults with department directors and managers on problems that can be solved through training.
- Facilitates training and orientation of new hires.
- Serves as an instructor for a variety of training programs when qualified.
- Coordinates external professional training if needed.
- Gathers and makes available appropriate training resources (e.g., books, DVDs, online resources) for professional development and personal use.
- Gathers and analyzes progress and results from training programs and prepares reports on findings.
- Ensure compliance with current healthcare regulations, medical laws, federal and state laws, and high ethical standards.

Education:

- Master's degree in education, health education, or human resource development.

Experience:

- Minimum five years of experience in health education management, with three years of experience in the healthcare industry.

Other Requirements:

- Must be available to have a mixed schedule of opening and closing the office and the ability to be flexible with schedule when needed.
- APTD certification from ADT.

Competency requirements:

Knowledge:

- Knowledge of instructional adult learning techniques and equipment, human resources development and quality management concepts.
- Knowledge of current trends and issues in professional training and development.
- Knowledge of how to identify education and training needs in healthcare setting and direct related program development and instruction.

Skills:

- Skill in program development and instruction.
- Skill in identifying trends in departments/programs and determining training impacts.
- Skill in developing cost-effective programs and facilitating cutting-edge training methods used by up-to-date training specialists.

Abilities:

- Ability to communicate effectively with all levels of employees; facilitate group processes and change.
- Ability to develop/make effective presentations and serve as a trainer when qualified.
- Ability to prioritize and coordinate multiple projects.

Equipment Operated:

- Standard office equipment including computers, fax machines, copiers, printers, telephones, etc.

Work Environment:

Position is in a well-lit office environment.
Occasional evening and weekend work.

Mental/Physical Requirements:

- Involves sitting approximately 90 percent of the day, walking or standing the remainder.
- Combination of sitting, standing, bending, light lifting and walking.
- Requires a full range of body motion including manual and finger dexterity and hand-eye coordination.
- Lifting up to 20 pounds.
- Requires corrected vision and hearing to a normal range.
- Requires the ability to manage stressful situations.
- Occasional stress from varying demands.

Disclaimer: This description is intended to provide only basic guidelines for meeting job requirements. Responsibilities, knowledge, skills, abilities, and working conditions may change as needs of the organization evolve and on an organization by organization basis.

Job Title: Business Development Specialist

Department: Administration

Immediate Supervisor Title: Practice Administrator

Job Supervisory Responsibilities: Designated
individuals in the accounting department

General Summary:

- Business development specialists are responsible for creating effective business plans for their company.
- They are also in charge of analyzing business processes and identifying opportunities to generate additional revenue.
- They research industries to find purchase patterns and emerging trends to recommend changes for their organization.
- Business development specialists also assess potential clients and provide development support, as well as act as a facilitator between executives and external contracting sources.
- They process large amounts of company data to make predictions and create detailed reports.
- Another of the specialist's main duties includes recommending changes to supply chain management as necessary.
- They also help implement growth strategies, participate in business meetings, and recommend changes to existing business practices to increase exposure and revenue.
- Business development specialists also assist with budget development and provide support for existing initiatives.

Essential Job Responsibilities:

- Quantifies business intelligence with economic models to evaluate new opportunities; presents findings clearly and makes recommendations for action.

- Assists with core business development activities, such as generating pitch decks and communicating with clients and competitors to better understand business trends.
- Seeks out new market insights and business opportunities through research and analysis.
- Establishes and maintains referral relationships.
- Maintains a database of physician contacts and referrals, tracking results and trends.
- Works with the marketing manager to develop new marketing strategies and new business.
- Works with the marketing communications specialist to develop new marketing materials.

Education:
- Bachelor's degree in marketing, communications, or business administration.

Experience:
- Minimum three years of experience in business development, preferably in the healthcare industry.

Other Requirements:
- Must be available to have a mixed schedule of opening and closing the office and the ability to be flexible with schedule when needed.
- MGMA certification.

Competency requirements:

Knowledge:
- Knowledge of and experience with [vendor-specific EHR] is preferred.
- Knowledge of Electronic Health Systems in any case
- Knowledge of Practice Management Systems

- Knowledge of proper phone etiquette and phone handling skills.
- Knowledge of organizational policies, procedures, and systems.
- Knowledge of office management techniques and practices.
- Knowledge of computer systems, programs, and applications.
- Knowledge of research methods and procedures sufficient to compile data and prepare reports.
- Knowledge of grammar, spelling, and punctuation.
- General knowledge of healthcare terminology preferred.
- Knowledge of purchasing, budgeting, and inventory control.

Skills:

- Skill in taking and transcribing dictation and in the operation of office equipment.
- This position requires strong working knowledge of managed care plans, insurance carriers, referrals and precertification procedures.
- Ability to communicate in English, both verbally and in writing.
- Additional languages preferred.
- CPT and ICD-10 coding abilities preferred.
- Must possess strong human relations, communication, problem solving, and organizational skills to interact with a variety of customers and personnel, both within and outside the institution.
- Must be able to work independently and in a team environment.
- Requires strong personal computer skills, communication skills, problem solving, continuous improvement and teaming skills.
- Maintains a broad knowledge of clinical, financial, and administrative systems/applications and processes.

- Serves as a resource on department and institutional initiatives; shares knowledge with customers and colleagues.
- Demonstrated verbal and written communication skills.

Abilities:

- Must maintain regular and acceptable attendance; may be required to work weekend, holiday or OT hours.
- Ability to establish and maintain effective working relationships with other employees and the public.
- Ability to work under pressure, communicate and present information.
- Ability to read, interpret, and apply clinic policies and procedures.
- Ability to identify problems, recommend solutions, organize and analyze information.
- Ability to establish priorities and coordinate work activities.
- Exposure to electronic health record preferred.
- Ability to work independently, be goal-directed and have strong organizational skills.
- Effectively multitask without compromising quality.
- Ability to comprehend and excel in both verbal and written communication, including proper telephone etiquette, face-to-face interactions, and electronic communications.
- Ability to communicate with individuals and small groups with credibility and confidence.
- Ability to handle difficult situations, remain calm under stress, manage emotional situations, display empathy and maintain positive communication during a rapidly changing/dynamic environment.
- Turn problems into opportunities by developing innovative and creative solutions.
- Demonstrate a friendly, positive attitude, display energy and drive in performing daily responsibilities.

- Must be flexible as well as easily adapt to a changing work environment which will require ongoing maintenance of job-related skills/activities.
- Must be willing to adjust work schedules in response to department or clinical needs.
- Able to manage and prioritize tasks simultaneously while working directly with patients who may exhibit diverse needs.

Equipment Operated:
- Standard office equipment including computers, fax machines, copiers, printers, telephones, etc.

Work Environment:
Position is in a well-lit office environment. Occasional evening and weekend work.

Mental/Physical Requirements:
- Involves sitting approximately 90 percent of the day, walking or standing the remainder.
- Combination of sitting, standing, bending, light lifting and walking.
- Requires a full range of body motion including manual and finger dexterity and hand-eye coordination.
- Requires corrected vision and hearing to a normal range.
- Requires the ability to manage stressful situations.
- Occasional stress from varying demands.

Disclaimer: This description is intended to provide only basic guidelines for meeting job requirements. Responsibilities, knowledge, skills, abilities, and working conditions may change as needs of the organization evolve and on an organization by organization basis.

Job Title: Chief Technology Officer

Department: Information Technology
Immediate Supervisor Title: Chief Executive Officer
Job Supervisory Responsibilities: IT department

General Summary:

A management position responsible for planning, directing, developing, and maintaining the medical practice's information technology, including computers, computer networks and servers, computer programs, telecommunications, Website, and other technologies.

Essential Job Responsibilities:

- Develops mission, plan, goals, policies, and budget for the Information Technologies department.
- Works with management team to identify strategic Information Technologies needs and establishes priorities for upgrades and modifications in line with clinic goals.
- Develops, recommends, coordinates, and implements new or revised procedures, policies, programs, and equipment to ensure Information Technologies effectiveness.
- Assists in correcting technical problems and issues as needed.
- Ensures that computer hardware, including all computers, fax machines, printer, copiers, etc., function properly on a daily basis.
- Develops and implements effective data backup and hardware security procedures and policies.

Education:

- Master's degree in computer science or information technology.

Experience:

- Minimum five years of experience in managing information technology in an office environment, preferably in the healthcare setting.

Competency requirements:

Knowledge:

- Knowledge of policies and procedures to manage operations and ensure effective patient care.
- Knowledge of the principles and practices of healthcare administration, fiscal management, and government regulations and reimbursements.
- Knowledge of Electronic Health Systems.
- Knowledge of Practice Management Systems.
- Knowledge of proper phone etiquette and phone handling skills.
- Knowledge of organizational policies, procedures, and systems.
- Knowledge of office management techniques and practices.
- Knowledge of computer systems, programs, and applications.
- Knowledge of research methods and procedures sufficient to compile data and prepare reports.
- Knowledge of grammar, spelling, and punctuation.
- General knowledge of healthcare terminology preferred.
- Knowledge of purchasing, budgeting, and inventory control.
- Knowledge of data analysis, systems design, problem identification, and medical data processing practice.
- Knowledge of computer and server hardware, software, and data communications including comparability and system configuration.
- Knowledge of basic programming languages.
- Knowledge of fiscal management.

Skills:

- Skill in using communication methods to elicit information, negotiate, resolve problems, and garner support.
- Skill over a broad range of functional information technology management.
- Skill in programming and project management if necessary to resolve critical problems, coordinate simultaneous efforts, recover from data loss, speed up development, and improve program efficiencies.
- Skill in exercising a high degree of initiative, judgment, and discretion.
- Skill in analyzing situations accurately and taking effective action.
- Skill in establishing and maintaining effective working relationships.
- Skill in organizing work, delegating and achieving goals and objectives.
- Skill in exercising judgment and discretion in developing, interpreting, and implementing departmental policies and procedures.
- Ability to communicate in English, both verbally and in writing.
- Additional languages preferred.
- Must possess strong human relations, communication, problem solving, and organizational skills to interact with a variety of customers and personnel, both within and outside the institution.
- Must be able to work independently and in a team environment.
- Requires strong personal computer skills, communication skills, problem solving, continuous improvement and teaming skills.
- Maintains a broad knowledge of clinical, financial, and administrative systems/applications and processes.

- Serves as a resource on department and institutional initiatives; shares knowledge with customers and colleagues.
- Demonstrated verbal and written communication skills.

Abilities:

- Ability to resolve conflicts productively.
- Ability to separate problems into components and recognize underlying patterns and processes.
- Ability to establish and maintain effective working relationships with other employees and the public.
- Ability to work under pressure, communicate and present information.
- Ability to read, interpret, and apply clinic policies and procedures.
- Ability to identify problems, recommend solutions, organize and analyze information.
- Ability to establish priorities and coordinate work activities.
- Exposure to electronic health record preferred.
- Ability to work independently, be goal-directed and have strong organizational skills.
- Effectively multitask without compromising quality.
- Ability to comprehend and excel in both verbal and written communication, including proper telephone etiquette, face-to-face interactions, and electronic communications.
- Ability to communicate with individuals and small groups with credibility and confidence.
- Ability to handle difficult situations, remain calm under stress, manage emotional situations, display empathy and maintain positive communication during a rapidly changing/dynamic environment.
- Turn problems into opportunities by developing innovative and creative solutions.
- Demonstrate a friendly, positive attitude, display energy and drive in performing daily responsibilities.

- Must be flexible as well as easily adapt to a changing work environment which will require ongoing maintenance of job-related skills/activities.
- Must be willing to adjust work schedules in response to department or clinical needs.
- Ability to be oriented to end-user needs.

Equipment Operated:

- Standard office equipment including computers, fax machines, copiers, printers, telephones, etc.

Work Environment:

Position is in a well-lit office environment. Occasional evening and weekend work.

Mental/Physical Requirements:

- Involves sitting approximately 90 percent of the day, walking or standing the remainder.
- Combination of sitting, standing, bending, light lifting and walking.
- Requires a full range of body motion including manual and finger dexterity and hand-eye coordination.
- Requires corrected vision and hearing to a normal range.
- Requires the ability to manage stressful situations.
- Occasional stress from varying demands.

Disclaimer: This description is intended to provide only basic guidelines for meeting job requirements. Responsibilities, knowledge, skills, abilities, and working conditions may change as needs of the organization evolve and on an organization by organization basis.

Job Title: Communications Specialist

Department: Information Technology

Immediate Supervisor Title: Chief Technology Officer

Job Supervisory Responsibilities:

General Summary:

A technical position responsible for the medical practice's telecommunications system including telephone system, voicemail, and conference calling arrangements.

Essential Job Responsibilities:

- Enhance patient experiences; optimizing company reputation.
- Ensure compliance with current healthcare regulations, medical laws, federal and state laws, and high ethical standards.
- Manages all telecommunications infrastructure including telephones, voice mail services, call forwarding options, conference calling, etc.
- Develops and maintains policies and procedures regarding telephones. Trains new hires on the communication system.
- Monitors and maintains the telecommunication system ensuring high performance.
- Diagnoses and resolves problems within the system.
- Troubleshoots and fixes employee's problems with phones and voice mail.

Education:

- Bachelor's degree in Information Technology or related field.
- Completion of a medical terminology course or successful completion within six months of employment.

Experience:

- Minimum two years of experience maintaining telecommunication systems, preferably in the healthcare setting.

Other Requirements:

- Must be available to have a mixed schedule of opening and closing the office and the ability to be flexible with schedule when needed.
- MGMA certification.

Competency requirements:

Knowledge:

- Knowledge of policies and procedures to manage operations and ensure effective patient care.
- Knowledge of telephones, voice lines, data lines, and voice mail.
- Knowledge of installation techniques of phone systems.
- Knowledge of current trends in telecommunications.

Skills:

- Skill in prioritizing tasks and project management.
- Skill in using customer service skills in dealing with employees.
- Skill in problem solving.
- Skill in exercising a high degree of initiative, judgment, and discretion.
- Skill in analyzing situations accurately and taking effective action.
- Skill in establishing and maintaining effective working relationships.
- Skill in organizing work, delegating and achieving goals and objectives.

Abilities:

- Ability to communicate effectively with all levels of employees.
- Ability to a team player with effective interpersonal skills.
- Ability to solve problems and work independently.
- Must maintain regular and acceptable attendance; may be required to work weekend, holiday or OT hours.
- Ability to establish and maintain effective working relationships with other employees and the public.
- Ability to work under pressure, communicate and present information.

Equipment Operated:

- Standard office equipment including computers, fax machines, copiers, printers, telephones, etc.
- Networked computers and servers and associated hardware.

Work Environment:

Position is in a well-lit office environment.
Occasional evening and weekend work.

Mental/Physical Requirements:

- Involves sitting approximately 90 percent of the day, walking or standing the remainder.
- Combination of sitting, standing, bending, light lifting and walking.
- Requires a full range of body motion including manual and finger dexterity and hand-eye coordination.
- Lifting up to 20 pounds.
- Requires corrected vision and hearing to a normal range.
- Requires the ability to manage stressful situations.
- Occasional stress from varying demands.

Disclaimer: This description is intended to provide only basic guidelines for meeting job requirements. Responsibilities, knowledge, skills, abilities, and working conditions may change as needs of the organization evolve and on an organization by organization basis.

Job Title: Computer Support Specialist

Department: Information Technology
Immediate Supervisor Title: Chief Technology Officer
Job Supervisory Responsibilities:

General Summary:

A position responsible for helping employees troubleshoot and fix computer-related problems.

Essential Job Responsibilities:

- Provides all employees troubleshooting services and support for all operating system-, application-, program-, and hardware-related problems.
- Works with the IT technical assistant to set up new computers.
- Collaborate with vendor or clinic IT engineers and software developers to select appropriate design solutions or ensure the compatibility of system components.
- Evaluate current or emerging technologies to consider factors such as cost, portability, compatibility, or usability.
- Maintains functionality of all computers and printers.
- Records and files all computer problems. Documents corrective actions taken.
- Assists in computer program training.

Education:

- High school diploma required;
- Bachelor's degree or higher or foreign equivalent in computer science, math, engineering, applied physics, or closely related field of study preferred.

Experience:

- Minimum two years of experience in computer support services, preferably in the healthcare industry.

Other Requirements:

- Must be available to have a mixed schedule of opening and closing the office and the ability to be flexible with schedule when needed.

Competency requirements:

Knowledge:

- Knowledge of and experience with [vendor-specific EHR] is preferred.
- Knowledge of Electronic Health Systems in any case.
- Knowledge of Practice Management Systems.
- Basic knowledge of TCP/IP networking.
- Demonstrated knowledge and skills operating Microsoft Active Directory in a large, complex organization.
- Demonstrated knowledge of security procedures for credential hygiene
- Knowledge of proper phone etiquette and phone handling skills.
- Knowledge of organizational policies, procedures, and systems.
- Knowledge of office management techniques and practices.
- Knowledge of computer systems, programs, and applications.
- Knowledge of grammar, spelling, and punctuation.
- General knowledge of healthcare terminology preferred.
- Knowledge of computer training principles and techniques.

Skills:

- Ability to communicate in English, both verbally and in writing.

- Additional languages preferred.
- Must possess strong human relations, communication, problem solving, and organizational skills to interact with a variety of customers and personnel, both within and outside the institution.
- Must be able to work independently and in a team environment.
- Requires strong personal computer skills, communication skills, problem solving, continuous improvement and teaming skills.
- Maintains a broad knowledge of clinical, financial, and administrative systems/applications and processes.
- Serves as a resource on department and institutional initiatives; shares knowledge with customers and colleagues.
- Demonstrated verbal and written communication skills.
- Skill in training variety of users on computer applications and programs.

Abilities:

- Must maintain regular and acceptable attendance; may be required to work weekend, holiday or OT hours.
- Ability to establish and maintain effective working relationships with other employees and the public.
- Ability to work under pressure, communicate and present information.
- Ability to take responsibility and accountability for own activities.
- Ability to read, interpret, and apply clinic policies and procedures.
- Ability to identify problems, recommend solutions, organize and analyze information.
- Ability to establish priorities and coordinate work activities.
- Exposure to electronic health record preferred.
- Ability to work independently, be goal-directed and have strong organizational skills.

- Effectively multitask without compromising quality.
- Ability to comprehend and excel in both verbal and written communication, including proper telephone etiquette, face-to-face interactions, and electronic communications.
- Ability to communicate with individuals and small groups with credibility and confidence.
- Ability to handle difficult situations, remain calm under stress, manage emotional situations, display empathy and maintain positive communication during a rapidly changing/dynamic environment.
- Turn problems into opportunities by developing innovative and creative solutions.
- Demonstrate a friendly, positive attitude, display energy and drive in performing daily responsibilities.
- Must be flexible as well as easily adapt to a changing work environment which will require ongoing maintenance of job-related skills/activities.
- Must be willing to adjust work schedules in response to department or clinical needs.
- Ability to clearly explain computer applications and programs in simple, user-friendly ways.
- Ability to effectively interact with all employees at all levels of computer understanding.

Equipment Operated:
- Standard office equipment including computers, fax machines, copiers, printers, telephones, etc.

Work Environment:
Position is in a well-lit office environment. Occasional evening and weekend work.

Mental/Physical Requirements:
- Involves sitting approximately 90 percent of the day, walking or standing the remainder.

Disclaimer: This description is intended to provide only basic guidelines for meeting job requirements. Responsibilities, knowledge, skills, abilities, and working conditions may change as needs of the organization evolve and on an organization by organization basis.

Job Title: .NET Developer Patient Online Services
Department: Information Technology
Immediate Supervisor Title: Chief Technology Officer
Job Supervisory Responsibilities:

General Summary:

A administrative position responsible for developing, communicating, installing, and maintaining databases while ensuring high security and ease of data availability.

Essential Job Responsibilities:

- Using knowledge of ASP.Net MVC, jQuery, DICOM, ESB, HL7, and MS SQL Server, design, architect, develop, and troubleshoot IT solutions for unique, complex, and innovative applications, system administration issues, and network concerns for proton therapy and upcoming critical programs currently in planning and development Clinic.
- Communicate with staff physicians and physicists to understand specific system and user requirements.
- Evaluate current or emerging technologies to consider factors such as cost, portability, compatibility, or usability.
- Document design specifications, installation instructions, and other system-related information.
- Work with Clinic Information Technology and Office of Information Security staff to implement and maintain current IT security best practices.
- Work with clinic and vendor staff to implement systems, integrate systems into clinic architecture, troubleshoot, and provide enhancement and bug fix feedback to vendors.

- Maintain pro-active monitoring systems and solutions to prevent and detect potential problems that would impact patient care or business continuity.
- Maintain Outcomes DataMart which aggregates patient treatment data across current and legacy systems allowing for research to compare cost and clinical effectiveness of proton versus traditional photon therapies.
- Coordinates with end users as to inputs and outputs are required, desired and superfluous.
- Works with department directors and managers to develop policies and procedures regarding databases and security of data.
- Ensures compliance with all database data and security of the data.
- Develops procedures and policies to ensure high performance and ease of access for all users.
- Designs and implements security and back-up systems for data recovery. Completes security audits to ensure that systems operate properly.

Education:

- Bachelor's degree or higher or foreign equivalent in computer science, information technology, or related field.

Experience:

- Minimum five years of experience of database administration, preferably in the healthcare industry.

Other Requirements:

- Must be available to have a mixed schedule of opening and closing the office and the ability to be flexible with schedule when needed.
- MGMA certification.

Competency requirements:

Knowledge:

- Knowledge of and experience with [vendor-specific EHR] is preferred.
- Knowledge of Electronic Health Systems in any case.
- Knowledge of Practice Management Systems.
- Basic knowledge of TCP/IP networking.
- Demonstrated knowledge and skills operating Microsoft Active Directory in a large, complex organization.
- Demonstrated knowledge of security procedures for credential hygiene
- Knowledge of proper phone etiquette and phone handling skills.
- Knowledge of organizational policies, procedures, and systems.
- Knowledge of office management techniques and practices.
- Knowledge of computer systems, programs, and applications.
- Knowledge of grammar, spelling, and punctuation.
- General knowledge of healthcare terminology preferred
- Knowledge of developing and building SQL databases.
- Knowledge of data security and recovery techniques.
- Knowledge of troubleshooting database problems.

Skills:

- Ability to communicate in English, both verbally and in writing.
- Additional languages preferred.
- Must possess strong human relations, communication, problem solving, and organizational skills to interact with a variety of customers and personnel, both within and outside the institution.
- Must be able to work independently and in a team environment.
- Skill in providing attention to detail and documentation.

- Skill in both oral and written communication.
- Skill in building effective working relationships.

Abilities:

- Must maintain regular and acceptable attendance; may be required to work weekend, holiday or OT hours.
- Ability to establish and maintain effective working relationships with other employees and the public.
- Ability to work under pressure, communicate and present information.
- Ability to take responsibility and accountability for own activities.
- Ability to communicate in a user-friendly, simple manner.
- Ability to solve problems effectively.
- Ability to be well organized and prioritize effectively.

Equipment Operated:

- Standard office equipment including computers, fax machines, copiers, printers, telephones, etc.

Work Environment:

Position is in a well-lit office environment. Occasional evening and weekend work.

Mental/Physical Requirements:

- Involves sitting approximately 90 percent of the day, walking or standing the remainder.
- Combination of sitting, standing, bending, light lifting and walking.
- Requires a full range of body motion including manual and finger dexterity and hand-eye coordination.
- Requires corrected vision and hearing to a normal range.
- Requires the ability to manage stressful situations.
- Occasional stress from varying demands.

Disclaimer: This description is intended to provide only basic guidelines for meeting job requirements. Responsibilities, knowledge, skills, abilities, and working conditions may change as needs of the organization evolve and on an organization by organization basis.

Job Title: IT Technical Assistant

Department: Information Technology
Immediate Supervisor Title: Chief Technology Officer
Job Supervisory Responsibilities:

General Summary:

Using knowledge of ASP.Net MVC, jQuery, DICOM, ESB, HL7, and MS SQL Server, design, architect, develop, and troubleshoot IT solutions for unique, complex, and innovative applications, system administration issues, and network concerns for proton therapy and upcoming critical programs currently in planning and development by the Department of Radiation Oncology at Clinic. Communicate with staff physicians and physicists to understand specific system and user requirements.

Provide advice on project costs, design concepts, or design changes.

Collaborate with vendor or Clinic IT engineers and software developers to select appropriate design solutions or ensure the compatibility of system components.

Evaluate current or emerging technologies to consider factors such as cost, portability, compatibility, or usability.

Document design specifications, installation instructions, and other system-related information.

Work with Clinic Information Technology and Office of Information Security staff to implement and maintain current IT security best practices.

Work with clinic and vendor staff to implement systems, integrate systems into clinic architecture, troubleshoot, and provide enhancement and bug fix feedback to vendors.

Maintain pro-active monitoring systems and solutions to prevent and detect potential problems that would impact patient care or business continuity.

Maintain, in conjunction with medical physics team, a GPU accelerated Monte-Carlo engine and interface for use in clinical practice which modifies the dose optimization algorithm to account for uncertainties in proton therapy delivery.

Maintain Gamma knife application and database which have been used over decades to produce an extremely productive pipeline of research articles for the Departments of Radiation Oncology and Neurosurgery.

Maintain Deviation from Standard Operation Procedure (DSOP) application which aggregates treatment events which fail to follow proper procedure and thus enhance patient care.

Maintain workflow for DICOM image archive which allows for the saving of decades of DICOM image and radiation therapy treatment data to a third-party archive allowing access to researchers and clinical users.

Maintain Outcomes DataMart which aggregates patient treatment data across current and legacy systems allowing for research to compare cost and clinical effectiveness of proton versus traditional photon therapies.

Role involves: CUDA, C++, Python, Bootstrap 3, Open Grid Scheduler, Windows, and Centos 6.9.

Work with the following tools and technologies: ASP.NET MVC 4, WebAPI, jQuery, Enterprise Framework, CUDA, C++, Python, Bootstrap 3, MS SQL Server, Merge DICOM toolkit, Open Grid Scheduler, Windows, Centos 6.9.

Coordinates with end users as to inputs and outputs are required, desired and superfluous.

Essential Job Responsibilities:

- Enhance patient experiences; optimizing company reputation.
- Ensure compliance with current healthcare regulations, medical laws, federal and state laws, and high ethical standards.

Education:

- Bachelor's degree or higher or foreign equivalent in Computer Science, Math, Engineering, Applied Physics, or closely related field of study.

Experience:

- The position requires 5 years (60 months) of experience as a Technical Specialist, Analyst Programmer or closely related field utilizing the following tools and technologies: C#, ASP.NET MVC, jQuery, DICOM, ESB, HL7 and MS SQL Server.
- All experience may be gained concurrently.

Other Requirements:

- Must be available to have a mixed schedule of opening and closing the office and the ability to be flexible with schedule when needed.
- MGMA certification.

Competency requirements:

Knowledge:

- Knowledge of and experience with [vendor-specific EHR] is preferred.
- Knowledge of Electronic Health Systems in any case.
- Knowledge of Practice Management Systems.
- Basic knowledge of TCP/IP networking.
- Demonstrated knowledge and skills operating Microsoft Active Directory in a large, complex organization.
- Demonstrated knowledge of security procedures for credential hygiene
- Knowledge of proper phone etiquette and phone handling skills.
- Knowledge of organizational policies, procedures, and systems.

- Knowledge of office management techniques and practices.
- Knowledge of computer systems, programs, and applications.
- Knowledge of grammar, spelling, and punctuation.
- General knowledge of healthcare terminology preferred.

Skills:

- Ability to communicate in English, both verbally and in writing.
- Additional languages preferred.
- Must possess strong human relations, communication, problem solving, and organizational skills to interact with a variety of customers and personnel, both within and outside the institution.
- Must be able to work independently and in a team environment.
- Requires strong personal computer skills, communication skills, problem solving, continuous improvement and teaming skills.
- Maintains a broad knowledge of clinical, financial, and administrative systems/applications and processes.
- Serves as a resource on department and institutional initiatives; shares knowledge with customers and colleagues.
- Demonstrated verbal and written communication skills.

Abilities:

- Must maintain regular and acceptable attendance; may be required to work weekend, holiday or OT hours.
- Ability to establish and maintain effective working relationships with other employees and the public.
- Ability to work under pressure, communicate and present information.
- Ability to take responsibility and accountability for own activities.

- Ability to read, interpret, and apply clinic policies and procedures.
- Ability to identify problems, recommend solutions, organize and analyze information.
- Ability to establish priorities and coordinate work activities.
- Exposure to electronic health record preferred.
- Ability to work independently, be goal-directed and have strong organizational skills.
- Effectively multitask without compromising quality.
- Ability to comprehend and excel in both verbal and written communication, including proper telephone etiquette, face-to-face interactions, and electronic communications.
- Ability to communicate with individuals and small groups with credibility and confidence.
- Ability to handle difficult situations, remain calm under stress, manage emotional situations, display empathy and maintain positive communication during a rapidly changing/dynamic environment.
- Turn problems into opportunities by developing innovative and creative solutions.
- Demonstrate a friendly, positive attitude, display energy and drive in performing daily responsibilities.
- Must be flexible as well as easily adapt to a changing work environment which will require ongoing maintenance of job-related skills/activities.
- Must be willing to adjust work schedules in response to department or clinical needs.
- Able to manage and prioritize tasks simultaneously while working directly with patients who may exhibit diverse needs.

Equipment Operated:

Standard office equipment including computers, fax machines, copiers, printers, telephones, etc.

Work Environment:

Position is in a well-lit office environment. Occasional evening and weekend work.

Mental/Physical Requirements:

- Involves sitting approximately 90 percent of the day, walking or standing the remainder.
- May need to lift up to 30 pounds.

Disclaimer: This description is intended to provide only basic guidelines for meeting job requirements. Responsibilities, knowledge, skills, abilities, and working conditions may change as needs of the organization evolve and on an organization by organization basis.

Job Title: Computer Programmer/ Analyst

Department: Information Technology
Immediate Supervisor Title: Chief Technology Officer
Job Supervisory Responsibilities:

General Summary:

Provides IT support for vended and custom applications, including resolving highly complex issues, and assists with data security, redundancy, and support in collaboration with more senior technical staff.

Conducts root-cause analysis by researching hardware environment and software application and system problems, works with colleagues and customers to resolve issues, documents resolution, and communicates resolution with customer.

Regularly reviews applications and makes modifications and/ or updates of a single system application or basic software and their associated hardware at multiple Clinic sites to ensure currency and functionality within the established environment.

Contributes to the design, development, implementation, and maintenance of custom system software, and/or the installation and maintenance of purchased systems software, as well as the configuration and support of hardware systems across the Clinic.

Coordinates with end users as to inputs and outputs are required, desired and superfluous.

Produces and maintains documentation such as systems requirements, designs, resource inventories and plans as requested. Interfaces routinely with colleagues who may be located at any of the Clinic practices to perform job responsibilities requiring virtual collaboration and partnership. May be required to provide 24/7 on-call support.

Essential Job Responsibilities:

- Enhance patient experiences; optimizing company reputation.
- Ensure compliance with current healthcare regulations, medical laws, federal and state laws, and high ethical standards.

Education:

- Bachelor's degree or higher or foreign equivalent in computer science, math, engineering, applied physics, or closely related field of study.
- OR, Associate degree and 5 years' professional experience in technical development.

Experience:

- The position requires 5 years (60 months) of experience as a Technical Specialist, Analyst Programmer or closely related field utilizing the following tools and technologies: C#, ASP.NET MVC, jQuery, DICOM, ESB, HL7 and MS SQL Server.
- All experience may be gained concurrently.

Other Requirements:

- Must be available to have a mixed schedule of opening and closing the office and the ability to be flexible with schedule when needed.

Competency requirements:

Knowledge:

- Knowledge of system design principles, software development methodologies, and computer programming.
- May interface with vendor support service groups or other external support teams to ensure proper

escalation during outages or periods of degraded system performance.

- Acts as a liaison to Clinic departments and vendors to adequately support the division's computing systems.
- Experience working in healthcare technology.
- Exposure to managing both custom developed and vendor-supplied applications.

Skills:

- Ability to communicate in English, both verbally and in writing.
- Additional languages preferred.
- Must possess strong human relations, communication, problem solving, and organizational skills to interact with a variety of customers and personnel, both within and outside the institution.
- Must be able to work independently and in a team environment.
- Requires strong personal computer skills, communication skills, problem solving, continuous improvement and teaming skills.
- Maintains a broad knowledge of clinical, financial, and administrative systems/applications and processes.
- Serves as a resource on department and institutional initiatives; shares knowledge with customers and colleagues.
- Demonstrated verbal and written communication skills.

Abilities:

- Must maintain regular and acceptable attendance; may be required to work weekend, holiday or OT hours.
- Ability to establish and maintain effective working relationships with other employees and the public.
- Ability to work under pressure, communicate and present information.
- Ability to take responsibility and accountability for own activities.

- Ability to read, interpret, and apply clinic policies and procedures.
- Ability to identify problems, recommend solutions, organize and analyze information.
- Ability to establish priorities and coordinate work activities.
- Exposure to electronic health record preferred.
- Ability to work independently, be goal-directed and have strong organizational skills.
- Effectively multitask without compromising quality.
- Ability to comprehend and excel in both verbal and written communication, including proper telephone etiquette, face-to-face interactions, and electronic communications.
- Ability to communicate with individuals and small groups with credibility and confidence.
- Ability to handle difficult situations, remain calm under stress, manage emotional situations, display empathy and maintain positive communication during a rapidly changing/dynamic environment.
- Turn problems into opportunities by developing innovative and creative solutions.
- Demonstrate a friendly, positive attitude, display energy and drive in performing daily responsibilities.
- Must be flexible as well as easily adapt to a changing work environment which will require ongoing maintenance of job-related skills/activities.
- Must be willing to adjust work schedules in response to department or clinical needs.
- Able to manage and prioritize tasks simultaneously while working directly with patients who may exhibit diverse needs.

Equipment Operated:

- Standard office equipment including computers, fax machines, copiers, printers, telephones, etc.

Work Environment:

Position is in a well-lit office environment. Occasional evening and weekend work.

Mental/Physical Requirements:

- Involves sitting approximately 90 percent of the day, walking or standing the remainder.
- May need to lift up to 30 pounds.

Disclaimer: This description is intended to provide only basic guidelines for meeting job requirements. Responsibilities, knowledge, skills, abilities, and working conditions may change as needs of the organization evolve and on an organization by organization basis.

Appendix B:
Sample Interview Questions

These are specific behavior-based questions for the different roles in financial management. Build on these to obtain the information needed to determine if the candidate has the skillset and abilities to address some of these common issues.

Standard Questions for Financial Management Positions

There are many specific questions for each job title; this is a sampling of questions that could work for the job titles in this category.

- How do you handle conflict in the workplace? Have you had situations in your past when you disagreed with your supervisor and how did you handle it?
- Do you have an elevator pitch? What's the biggest challenge in your role? How do you know you're successful?
- Customer Service (any role though) – Tell me about a time when you weren't successful in providing good

customer service. What did you learn and what would you do differently?

- Success – how do you know when you've been successful in your role?
- How do you explain what you do to a 5-year old?
- You're talking with a coworker or patient and you notice a mistake on your materials, how do you handle this? What do you say?
- Tell me about a time when you've made decisions and afterward regretted it.

Specific Questions for Financial Management Positions

- CFO
  - How do you handle conflict in the workplace? Have you had situations in your past when you disagreed with the CEO and how did you handle it?
  - What are the performance indicators you monitor every month?
  - Tell me about your most productive time in your past employment.
  - How do you know you're successful in your role as CFO?
  - Tell me about how you forecast for the organization
- Chief Technology Officer
  - How do you monitor for cyber-attacks?
  - What concerns do you have regarding security and ransomware?
  - What is the most significant security threat that you've dealt with and how did you resolve it?
  - What's your background with HIPAA?
  - How do you stay current with the world of every changing technology?
  - What systems and platforms have you supported? Explain your philosophy and normal organizational structure.

- What are the pros and cons of outsourcing some of your technology?
- Human Resources Director/Manager
    - Do you have an HR philosophy or mission? Tell me about it.
    - Have you had a "seat at the table" previously? If not, why not?
    - How do you stay on top of current legal and employment rules and regulations?
    - What type of conflict have you had to handle between managers and staff members in the past?
- Accounting Clerk
    - Tell me about your experience and comfort with accounting software and technology?
    - How do you confirm accuracy and efficiency when performing data entry?
    - What do you enjoy most about your work as the accounting clerk and why?
    - What's your experience with spreadsheets and databases?
    - How do you balance when your numbers are off?
- Accounting Manager/Controller
    - Tell me about your experience and comfort with accounting software and technology?
    - What types of audit measures do you use?
    - What systems have you used in the past?
    - How do you reconcile accounts? What do you do when your financials are off – walk me through it.
    - How do you do a month end close?
    - Have you handled budgeting in the past? Tell me about your process.
    - What reporting structure do you work best in? (CFO, administrator)
- Credit Manager
    - Monitoring the A/R Aging report is one of the responsibilities, how do you determine if there are

going to be potential payment issues? How do you resolve?

- How do you reconcile the accounts? What timeframes do you do this?
- Have you worked with claims administrators and A/R collections previously? What do you find is challenging in that role?
- Why do you want this position in this practice?

- Payroll Administrator
  - What programs/companies have you worked with to handle payroll in the past?
  - How have you worked with HR in the past?
  - How do you audit your work and the work of your payroll clerks?
  - Tell me about a time when you've had a payroll error and an employee has been overpaid, what did you do? How was it handled?
  - What are the rules/laws associated with paying an employee their final paycheck?
  - What's your year-end process?

- Payroll Clerk
  - What programs have you used to process payroll?
  - What do you do with an unclaimed payroll checks?
  - Tell me about a time when you've had a payroll error and an employee has been overpaid, what did you do? How was it handled?
  - What are the rules/laws associated with paying an employee their final paycheck?
  - How do you handle employees who tell you their check is wrong?

- Senior Accountant
  - Walk me through the process for month end close.
  - Preparing month-end banking reconciliations is a tedious process. What do you like about it? What don't you like about it?

- o Tell me about preparing an actual to budget variance analysis.
- o What is your budgeting preparation process?
- o What's your involvement in past audits?
- Benefits specialist
  - o Working with payroll can prove difficult, how do you handle the day-to-day communication? What happens with a breakdown in communication with payroll?
  - o Walk me through how you reconcile benefits and how often do you do that?
  - o Have you negotiated benefit contracts previously? What is the thing you wish you could improve upon in the future when doing so? If not, how would you learn how to do that?
  - o What's the difficult part about providing benefits to the staff?
- Compensation Specialist
  - o How do you know if we're competitive in our market?
  - o How often do you feel we should be doing competitive market analysis?
  - o What type of systems have you worked with previously?
  - o Have you presented to senior leadership before?
  - o What is payroll compression?
  - o We just found out our top nurse is leaving us; how would you recommend we counter-offer?
- Recruiting Specialist
  - o Walk me through the process of how you manage recruitment activities.
  - o How do you source candidates – what methods?
  - o What do you feel most practices could add to their recruitment?

- You have two great candidates, equal in every way, what do you do to make your final decision? How do you coach the hiring manager?
- What type of pre-screening activities do you employ?
- What are your career aspirations?
- As you walked in here for an interview, what would you change about this process?
- Training Specialist
  - How do you determine the staff is effectively trained for their position?
  - After review of the training programs, you realize there is a gap, walk me through what you would do to implement a new training program.
  - How do adults learn? What do you think is the most challenging thing about training adults?
  - We need new competency-based curriculum, what would you do first to design this new program?
  - What's the best training you ever received and why?
- Business Development Specialist
  - Do you have a customer strategy that you use?
  - Tell me about times you have been successful and when you haven't. What's the difference and what did you learn?
  - The company's strategy for business development includes creating an incentive program, what do you think about that?
  - How do you track leads and work with them?
  - What do you like about being a business development person?
  - What are your career aspirations?
- Communications Specialist
  - What does this title mean to you?
  - How do you handle negative communications? Walk me through a scenario you had to communicate difficult information.

- ○ Have you tracked ROI of your communication program? What did you do to do this? How? What were your outcomes? What would you do differently here?
- Computer Support Specialist
  - ○ Share an experience where you helped a user or customer solve a difficult hardware or software problem.
  - ○ Walk me through your process for troubleshooting an issue using a real world example.
  - ○ What is the difference between RAS and UPN servers?
  - ○ A user tells you their computer has been slow. Troubleshoot this for me.
- Database Administrator
  - ○ This position may have a lot of stress and pressure handling the various programs/databases. How do you handle that on a daily basis? What do you do to take care of yourself?
  - ○ Tell me about the programs you've used in the past? Which ones do you like and enjoy using?
  - ○ How have you/what have you don't to - develop/ implement database changes in the past to improve performance?
- IT Technical Assistant
  - ○ A user tells you their computer has been slow. Troubleshoot this for me.
  - ○ Share an experience where you helped a user or customer solve a difficult hardware or software problem.
  - ○ This is a busy office, walk me through how you prioritize when two staff members need help at the same time.
  - ○ What's the hardest part about manning the help desk?

- Program Analyst
  - This work involves ensuring optimization of resources, walk me through your assessment techniques.
  - When you identify key issues with a program that are inhibiting financial improvements, what do you do to share this information?
  - Tell me about how you best work to analyze a program.
  - Have you experienced when you negatively rated a program and the company did it anyway? How do you handle? If not, how would you handle?

About the Authors

Penny M. Crow, MS, SHRM-SCP, RHIA, is a nationally recognized executive with progressive senior leadership experience in a wide range of healthcare organizations. As an RHIA, she has a successful track record in health information management, revenue cycle, risk management and quality improvement. Her MS in I-O Psychology, has fueled her passion about working with leaders to develop strategic thinking skills.

Christine Kalish, MBA, CMPE, is a senior executive and trusted healthcare advisor with deep experience in ambulatory care and academic medicine. She is a thought leader and strategist for emerging and expanding healthcare organizations. For more than thirty years, Kalish has been leading organizations and teams to develop critical infrastructure and growth planning to improve operations, workflow, human resources and revenue cycle. She continually searches for innovative ways to assist her clients so they can deliver quality care for the populations they serve.

Sharon Z. Ginchansky, MAOM, is a consultant specializing in leadership and organizational change. Her career spans more than twenty-five years of operational and human resources experience working as an executive in the healthcare field.

Contributor: Summer Humphreys, MBA